THE Y'S WAY
TO A
HEALTHY BACK

THE Y'S WAY TO A HEALTHY BACK

ALEXANDER MELLEBY

Former National Director
YMCA Healthy Back Program

WITH A FOREWORD BY

HANS KRAUS, M.D.

New Century Publishers, Inc.,

Book design by Tere LoPrete

Printing Code
19 20 21 22

Library of Congress Cataloging in Publication Data
Melleby, Alexander.
  The Y's way to a healthy back.
  Bibliography: p.
  Includes index.
  1. Backache—Prevention. 2. Exercise therapy. 3. YMCA. I. YMCA.
II. Title.
RD768.M43   1982   617'.56062   82-14474
ISBN 0-8329-0252-7
ISBN 0-8329-0147-4 (pbk.)

CONTENTS

v

FOREWORD

For the millions who suffer low back pain, regardless of age, height, weight, or sex, this book is the way to relief in most cases. It is based upon the largest and most successful program of its kind in the world—the *Y's Way to a Healthy Back*—a six-week course, offered by YMCAs throughout the United States, Canada, and Australia. It is equally effective and usable by individuals and groups at home or elsewhere when its easy, relaxing exercises are followed in simple word instruction, illustrated by drawings.

Since the program began in 1974, more than 150,000 people have taken it. A recent study of 13,000 of those who have gone through the program, the largest statistical study ever done on sufferers of low back pain, shows that 80% of them experienced significant relief or total elimination of pain upon completion of the course. As a physician specializing in physical medicine, I have had the opportunity to see many patients with low back problems. I have also been closely associated with the *Y's Way to a Healthy Back* program from its beginnings.

In the early 1970s, Alexander Melleby asked me to form a medical committee to assist him in his work as Director of physical fitness programs for the YMCA of Greater New York. He had already an excellent reputation in his field, and I gladly con-

sented. It was soon apparent that Al was not only very knowledgeable, but an extraordinarily efficient and capable organizer
and administrator. We ran a few pilot sessions and gradually
established the exercise sequence now used in the *Y's Way to a
Healthy Back* program.

Thanks to Al's unceasing efforts the program has expanded
rapidly. At first I participated in all sessions for training of Y
"back pain teachers" and I found myself moving around the
United States like a traveling salesman. Soon an acceptable two-
day format of practical and theoretical teaching was established
and Al took over most of the work alone, giving me the chance to
enjoy my weekends at home instead of spending them in Ys all
over the country.

The *Y's Way to a Healthy Back* program is now firmly
established nationally and is growing rapidly both here and
abroad. This official course book, solidly based on safe medical
practice, will be of immediate and lasting value to those con-
cerned with low back pain. A chief ingredient of that value will be
the satisfaction of having relieved one's own back problems
through the use of this book, either alone or by participation in
the Y's healthy back program.

HANS KRAUS, M.D.

ACKNOWLEDGMENTS

The author would be remiss if he did not recognize three individuals and two groups of highly motivated YMCA professionals, and the National YMCA Committee of Medical Consultants, all of whom in one way or another carefully nurtured the Healthy Back program and brought it to its present state of pre-eminence.

First and foremost, this book would not have been possible had it not been for Hans Kraus, M.D., who initially gave me the program.

Second, the National Committee of Medical Consultants performed a major role in establishing Healthy Back program guidelines and policies to make sure that the entire effort met the highest possible standards of safety. I am most indebted again, to Hans Kraus, M.D., Committee Chairman, and William R. Bridges, M.D., Chairman, Dept. of Neurosurgery, Mobile Infirmary, Mobile, Alabama; C. Christopher Carruthers, M.D., Orthopedic Surgeon, Ottawa, Ontario, Canada; Sawnie R. Gaston, M.D., Orthopedic Surgeon, New York, New York; James P. McCarthy, Esquire, Attorney-at-Law, New York, New York; Willibald Nagler, M.D., Chief of Department of Physical Medicine, New York Hospital, New York, New York; Richard Traum, Ph.D., Behavioral Scientist, New York, New York; Herbert Walker, M.D., Psychiatric Medicine, New York, New York; and, Leon J. Warshaw, M.D., Occupational Medicine, New York, New York.

Third, I would like to offer special tribute to a group of YMCA professional health and physical educators who have expertly trained more than 3,000 local YMCA instructors during the past six years. Members of this group have played the key role in the rapid dissemination of the program throughout their respective countries. In the United States they are Jerry Beavers, San Jose, California; Charles Brown, Helena, Montana; Sam Brown, Glendale, California; Robert Calhoun, Seattle, Washington; Dan Carroll, Newport News, Virginia; Fred Cooper, Middletown, Ohio; Michael Cronin, Portland, Oregon; William Dunsworth, Orlando, Florida; Larry Garvin, Butler, Pennsylvania; Robert Glover, New York, New York; Robert Grenfell, San Diego, California; William Gregoire, Albuquerque, New Mexico; Glenn Gress, Fargo, North Dakota; Larry Hall, Dallas, Texas; Robert Hansen, Denver, Colorado; Paul Harvey, Quincy, Massachusetts; Dee Howell, Rome, New York; Stephen Kaye, Mobile, Alabama; Robert Laundy, Grantham, New Hampshire; John Mahurin, Mississippi State, Mississippi; Kenneth McGartlin, Memphis, Tennessee; Richard Moeller, Kansas City, Missouri; Marjorie Murphy, Chicago, Illinois; John Neumann, Springfield, Massachusetts; Faulds Orchard, Northbrook, Illinois; Betty Re', Waterville, Maine; Paula Reeder, Houston, Texas; Steven Ross, St. Louis, Missouri; Peggy Rude, Washington, D.C.; Jeff Sadowsky, Detroit, Michigan; James Scott, Findlay, Ohio; Steven Seiss, Rochester, New York; William Smith, Los Angeles, California; Greg Steel, Redlands, California; Sally Stewart, New York, New York; Michael Waldron, Harrisburg, Pennsylvania; Richard Webster, Minneapolis, Minnesota; Harold Welsh, Pittsburgh, Pennsylvania; and Brad Zerr, Berwyn, Pennsylvania.

The Canadian training team consisted of Robert Bonany, Sault Ste. Marie, Ontario; Rene DuPuis, Winnipeg, Manitoba; John Foster, London, Ontario; Claude McKenny, Ottawa, Ontario; Hartmut Rosenfeld, London, Ontario; Orazio Scaldaferri, Vancouver, British Columbia; Keith Simison, Windsor, Ontario; and Marty Snelling of Toronto, Ontario.

Instructor–Trainers for Australia are Joseph Brent and Diane Morgan of the Sydney YMCA, and Bruce Meakins of the Perth YMCA.

Instructor–Trainers in Japan are Osamu Kamiyama and Yasuhiko Iwase of the Tokyo YMCA.

Four, grateful appreciation is accorded to the thousands of YMCA instructors who carefully followed and taught the plan, bringing relief to tens of thousands of backache sufferers. Their willingness and patience in gathering data enabled Richard Traum, Ph.D., to conduct the largest study of its kind ever done on back pain.

Five, my wife Barbara proved that love transends all boundaries by providing hundreds of unpaid hours in keeping together the overall administration functions of the program. I know full well that without her volunteer efforts the Y's Way To A Healthy Back program would not have succeeded, and to her I am profoundly indebted.

Last but not least, I would like to thank Robert H. Boyle, a former back pain sufferer, for his editorial advice.

Alexander Melleby

To my parents

CHAPTER

1

You and Your Low Back Pain

If you suffer from low back pain, be glad that you've picked up this book and started reading it. Please read on, because it can be a life-saver for you, no matter what your age, sex, weight, or height. This book is based on the largest and most successful program of its kind in the world, the Y's Way to a Healthy Back program, a six-week course offered throughout the year at YMCAs in the United States, Canada, Australia, and Japan.

If you live near a Y that offers the Healthy Back program, I urge you to enroll. If you do not live near a Y offering the program or otherwise find it inconvenient to attend, use this book. Pay careful attention to the methods and procedures detailed here and follow them as instructed. As a matter of precaution, obtain approval from your physician before you start doing any exercises, simple as they may seem.

Although millions of people suffer from low back pain, it is not the baffling malady it is sometimes portrayed to be. Much available medical evidence clearly shows that more than 80 percent of all cases of low back pain are caused by weak and/or tense muscles, and *not* by organic lesions, such as vertebral disc disease, rheumatoid arthritis, benign or malignant tumors, infection, or fracture. I discuss the medical evidence at length in Chapter 14, but it is important that you know that weak and/or tense muscles are responsible for the great majority of all cases of low back pain. Thus, as bad as your back pain may be, the chances are better than 80 out of 100 that you can be helped by doing the exercises given in this book. These exercises, described in week-by-week sequence in Chapters 4 through 9, are designed to make your key postural muscles strong and flexible. That is the key to success in dealing with the vast majority of cases of low back pain.

I can say this with absolute confidence as the National Director of the Y's Way to a Healthy Back program. Since the Y began offering the program to the public in 1974, more than 150,000 people have taken it. Every year, each Y instructor giving the program is required to submit to our national office before-and-after survey forms filled out by the members of one class. We do this to keep track of the effectiveness of the program. In March of 1982, Richard Traum, Ph.D., a behavioral scientist who is President of PersonnelMetrics, Inc. in New York City and a member of the Y's Medical Advisory Board, completed a computer study of all the survey forms in our records. All told, forms had been filled out by 13,365 people across the country. Dr. Traum eliminated 1,556 of these forms simply because those who filled them out had not answered all 11 questions designed to measure pain. That left 11,809 subjects, and their answers were then fed into the PersonnelMetrics computer. The results: 9,532 people, or 80.7 percent, experienced improvement, while 2,277, or 19.3 percent did not. I know of no organizational approach that can match that figure of success. The study also showed that women composed 52 percent of the participants, men 48 percent. The average age of the participants was 49, and on average they had experienced back pain or discomfort for 8.1 years. The study is the largest ever done anywhere on sufferers of low back pain.

Recently, I began a follow-up study of 161 people who have continued to do the Y's Healthy Back exercises since they completed the program two and a half years ago. A total of 31 percent reported that they have had *complete* elimination of pain, 46 percent that they have had *much less* pain, and 23 percent that they have had *less* pain. One of the questions asked in the follow-up survey was, "How much money have you actually saved on medical bills while you have been taking this program?" Of 50 who responded, the average annual saving was $277.10. Fifty-five respondents indicated that before they began the Y's Way to a Healthy Back program they had lost a number of days from work over the course of a year. The total number of days lost by this group was 614, which cost them or their employers $61,400 in earnings and benefits. After taking the program and continuing with the exercises, the same 55 respondents reported losing a total of only 47 work days in a year. That's a saving of $56,700. It is exactly because of this kind of saving that numerous companies and government agencies have adopted the Y's Way to a Healthy Back program. Some of the largest insurance companies in the United States will actually pay policyholders to complete the course.

If your physician gives you approval to do the exercises in this book, take heart. Again, the chances are overwhelming that your low back pain is caused by weak and/or tense muscles, and that by the time you've finished with this book you'll be able to live a normal life without fear of another crippling attack. More than that, you'll probably be able to live life to the fullest and enjoy it to the utmost. At the Y, we're inundated with letters from people who took the program and are happy at last to be free of pain and worry. Some were in appalling shape and of desperate mind when they came to us. Here, for example, is the case of Peter B., a 40-year-old businessman. For almost a year before he entered the program, Mr. B. suffered from low back pain and sciatica. As the months wore on, he began to have increasing difficulty walking and sleeping. He had to give up normal chores and soon the pain intensified to the point where he suffered around the clock. "Before long I involuntarily worked myself into what I now know to be the very depressing and typical attitude of the back pain sufferer—that I would forever have low back pain," Mr. B. wrote. "In a period of seven months, I saw a chiropractor, an osteopath, a neurosurgeon and two orthopedic surgeons. With the exception of the chiropractor, each had a similar diagnosis: a disc out of place, and each recommended surgery, with a mere 30 percent chance of correction.

"By December," Mr. B. continued, "the pain became so

intense that I was unable to work and was rendered practically immobile. I was convinced that surgery was the only avenue left open to me. I went into the hospital for tests, and when I came out I read a feature story in the Sunday paper about the Y's Way to a Healthy Back program. I decided to hold off on surgery and take the program. What did I have to lose? I got into the program and by the fourth class I began to notice less pain. I still had a bit of pain when I finished the course two months ago, but now after continuing all the exercises on my own, I can state that *all* pain that I previously felt in my back and down the leg has disappeared completely. Not only am I able to do all the garden and lawn work as well as I did before, I have painted the house and done other chores, gone swimming and taken long vigorous walks, all activities that were unthinkable several months ago."

Two years later, Peter B. wrote, "I have performed the exercises every day for 19 months, and as a result I am able to perform any physical task without discomfort or fear of back pain. A day of unusual or strenuous work is not followed by soreness or discomfort. I eat better, sleep better, and have a general excellent sense of well-being. Each week I walk between 15 to 20 miles, sheer enjoyment I did not realize was there all along waiting for me. My sincere hope is that anyone who experiences back pain will enroll in the Y's Healthy Back program and dedicate himself or herself to the regular performance of the daily exercises. I feel so confident that many people can benefit from it as I have."

Mr. B. is not alone. Here is a letter from Kathryn Z., a 60-year-old woman who completed the Y's Healthy Back course. She titled her letter, "New Freedoms," and under this heading wrote:

"The first benefit—and to me the most important—was my freedom from fear of injuring my troublesome back.

"Having suffered about 25 years with 'a bad back,' I have known the agony of a pinched nerve, a pulled muscle, excruciating lower back pain. Having been treated in various ways—hospitalization, traction, machines, etc.—no one had ever offered any suggestions on how to *prevent* occurrence and recurrence of this dilemma. Therefore, I lived in fear that my next move could send me back to the hospital.

"Having confidence that the Y's program of exercise was safe gave me new hope that at last I was doing something positive about my problem.

"The next 'new freedom' I enjoyed was the freedom of movement. Without even realizing it, I found myself able to do things much more easily. Household chores that had me grunting and groaning could now be done with greater ease—even personal care, such as cutting my toenails, was accomplished easier.

"A very important new freedom was the easing of tension in my daily work, even in driving the car. A very beneficial side effect of learning how to relax—or becoming aware of relaxing—was in sleeping better at night.

"I feel a deep debt of gratitude to our Y instructor. Her understanding, her ability to help each and every one in the class, her willingness and eagerness to listen to individual problems, and her masterful control of us as a group are all very commendable.

"The benefits of this program will carry on in my life. I consider the Y's Way to a Healthy Back program a turning point, a new way of life!"

Mrs. Z.'s problem was caused by weak and tense muscles, but I might note here that even people who have undergone back surgery have benefited from the Y's Healthy Back exercises. Dr. William Bridges, a noted neurosurgeon in Mobile, Alabama, says, "I refer all my patients who have lumbar disc operations to the Healthy Back program, with most individuals obtaining excellent results."

CHAPTER

2

The Kraus–Weber Tests

If you suffer or have suffered from low back pain and like most people, have no organic lesions, there is a very easy method to find out why. You can take the six Kraus–Weber Tests described in this chapter. They are designed to test the strength and flexibility of the key muscle groups in your body. They reveal whether or not your muscles have the necessary strength and flexibility to handle your weight and height. Anyone can take them, regardless of age, weight or height, but do not take them if you are currently in pain.

The six tests were devised by Dr. Hans Kraus, an outstanding physician and authority in the field of physical medicine and rehabilitation, and Dr. Sonja Weber, a former colleague in the Department of Physical Therapy at Columbia Presbyterian Medical Center in New York City. I shall have more to say about Drs. Kraus and Weber and their important research and clinical findings in Chapter 14, but meanwhile, after getting your doctor's approval, take the tests to see why you have trouble.

In the Y's Way to a Healthy Back program, the instructor helps you take the Kraus–Weber Tests, but you can take them yourself if you can get a friend or family member to assist you as directed. When you are ready to take the tests, be sure that you are comfortable. Where appropriate, do the tests on an exercise mat or very firm mattress. Do *not* do them lying down on a hard floor. When you take the tests, make sure that you are comfortable. Take off your shoes and socks and strip down to your underclothes, or wear clothing that permits you to move freely and easily. Here is the first of the six tests.

Kraus–Weber Test No. 1

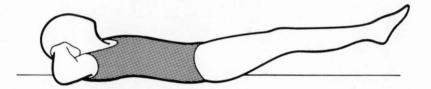

Position yourself comfortably on the floor, resting on your back. Your legs should be out straight, with ankles touching. Place your hands behind your neck. Now raise both feet (keeping knees straight) so that your heels are about 10 inches from the floor. You pass this test if you can hold your legs in this position for 10 seconds. This test measures minimum strength of hip flexor muscles.

Kraus–Weber Test No. 2

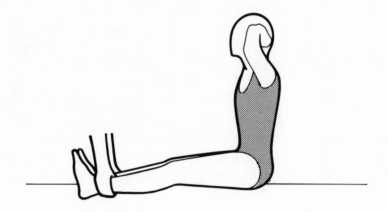

From this same position you now place your hands at the sides of your head. Make sure that someone is holding down your legs at the ankles as shown. Now roll up into a sit-up position. If you can complete the sit up, you have passed this test, which measures the combined strength of your hip flexors and abdominal muscles.

Kraus–Weber Test No. 3

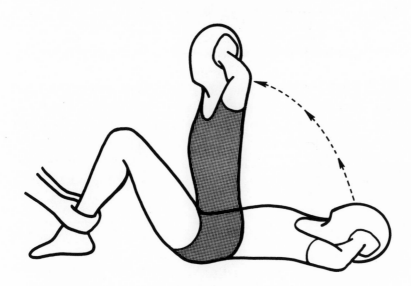

Again, lie flat on your back and place your hands at the sides of your head. Now bend both knees so that the heels are as close to the buttocks as possible without putting a strain on the knees. Your assistant should hold your ankles down. Now roll up into a sit-up position. If you can do the sit up, you pass the test. This measures the strength of your abdominal muscles.

Kraus–Weber Test No. 4

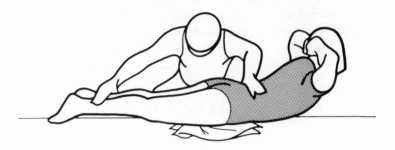

Roll over onto your stomach. Place a couple of pillows under the middle of your hips. Place your hands behind your neck. Your assistant should steady your body by placing one hand on the small of your back and the other hand at a point just above the heels. Now lift your upper body just enough to clear the floor and hold it steady for 10 seconds. If you can hold it for 10 seconds, you pass the test. This is a measure of the strength of your upper back muscles.

Kraus–Weber Test No. 5

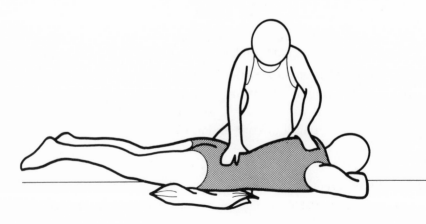

From this same position, rest your forehead on your hands as illustrated. Be sure to keep the pillows under your hips. This time have your assistant stabilize your body by placing one hand on your shoulders and the other hand on the small of the back. Keep your legs straight at the knees and raise both legs from the hips just enough to clear the floor and hold this position steady for 10 seconds. If you can hold this position for 10 seconds, you have passed this test, which measures the strength of your lower back muscles.

Kraus–Weber Test No. 6

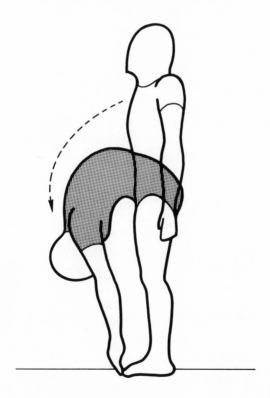

Stand erect, legs together, with your ankles touching each other. Relax at the shoulders, and place your chin on your chest.

Bend over and slowly reach toward the floor without bending your knees. See if you can touch the floor with your middle finger without straining. If you touch the floor, you have passed this test, which measures the flexibility of your back and the muscles in the backs of your legs. If you were unable to touch the floor, it is because you have lost the stretchability of these muscles which have become shortened over time. Inability to touch the floor also reflects tension in these muscles.

If you have failed any of the Kraus–Weber tests you now know why. It is because of the inability of those muscles that failed the test to support the body properly. Our records show that 61 percent of those entering the Y's Way to a Healthy Back program fail Kraus–Weber Test No. 6. They also show that 48 percent fail Kraus–Weber Test No. 3.

In the event that you are the unusual person who has had low back pain in the past but can pass all six Kraus–Weber Tests now, don't get the idea that you're Superman or Wonder Woman. As Dr. Kraus has stressed, these are *minimum* physical tests. If you pass all of them, it means that you have sufficient strength and flexibility to handle your own weight and height. But you can improve your muscular strength and flexibility by doing the exercises described in Chapters 4 through 11. If you play sports, you will find that these exercises will not only help to improve your performance but also serve as a preventive against athletic injuries.

Finally, those of you who have not had low back pain, but who have failed one or more of the six Kraus–Weber Tests, are not in the shape you should be in, and you are prime candidates for low back pain. Read on, so that you do not fall victim to this widespread and unnecessary malady.

CHAPTER

3

The Rationale of the Y's Exercise Program

The exercises that you will do for your back begin in the next chapter, but before you embark on them, I would like to describe their rationale. It's important that you know and understand fully the medical concepts behind them, because these exercises are different from any offered to the public today. They are also the most successful, and I want you to appreciate the reasons why they have been so successful.

First, the exercises in the Y's program fall into three different categories. These categories are designed to (1) relax your muscles, (2) make them flexible, and (3) strengthen them.

The relaxation exercises are used at the beginning and end of each and every exercise session. Relaxation is tremendously important. If you are unable to relax, you can't do anything beneficial for your muscles. The relaxation exercises will make you relax without your knowing it, and when your muscles relax, you will find that the inner tensions that caused your muscles to be tight will ebb and disappear. Moreover, the relaxation exercises will literally influence your mental state for the better, because your muscles have a way of working on the mind. The relaxation exercises give you triple benefits. One, they release muscle tension, which is frequently the root cause of back and neck discomfort. Two, by so doing, they help prepare you to do the stretching or flexibility exercises that follow, because it is difficult to stretch muscles that are tense and stiff. It is a physiological fact that a relaxed muscle will stretch and lengthen more easily than a tense muscle will. Three, the relaxation exercises will not only help reduce muscle tension, they also assist in reducing any muscle strain and soreness that you might suffer.

After you have done the relaxation exercises, your muscles are ready to do the stretching or flexibility exercises. By stretching and making your muscles more flexible, you lengthen your key postural muscles. These stretching exercises help you overcome muscle rigidity, and this in turn allows you to handle your body more efficiently. If your muscles are stiff, you can't move easily and you risk injury. You can see this for yourself if you are underexercised, especially if you are getting on in years. If you're 60 years old, you can't pop out of an armchair as readily as your teen-aged grandchild can because your muscles "jell" or stiffen more quickly with age. You have to stretch before you can move easily. An important point to bear in mind: all the flexibility exercises are specially arranged in sequence so that they prepare you for the more demanding exercises that follow, in much the same way that the relaxation exercises prepare you for the stretching exercises.

Now, a word about the strengthening exercises. They are designed only to strengthen your abdominal muscles. There is sound reason for this. Weak abdominal muscles are by far a more direct cause of back pain weakness than any other muscle group. In fact, there are so few people with weak back muscles that we do not even include exercises for them in the program. That may seem odd, but weak abdominal muscles are truly the biggest villain in causing back pain. Let me give you an example, and when you think about it, you'll say, "That's right." The example is a case history of a young mother whom I'll call Jan. Before she became pregnant, she was in excellent condition. She played tennis regularly, but when she knew she was going to have a baby, she gave up playing. Pregnancy put a strain on her abdominal muscles. It weakened them, and she did not know it. After she gave birth and came home from the hospital, she had to bend over the crib to look after her daughter, and because her abdominal muscles were weak, she had to overload the back muscles. One afternoon when she straightened up after changing diapers, she felt a sudden stab of pain in her lower back. The pain would not go away, and her husband had to look after their daughter over the weekend. By Monday, Jan felt better, but when she went to pick up the baby, the pain struck again, and this time her husband had to stay home for most of the week while she was immobilized in bed. Fortunately for Jan, she went to see her physician who put her on the exercise program the Y gives, and the back pain disappeared after she had strengthened her abdominal muscles.

Like the flexibility exercises, the abdominal strengthening exercises of the Healthy Back program are specially arranged in sequence, and each succeeding abdominal strengthing exercise is a bit more demanding than the previous one.

Now that I've explained the medical rationale behind the relaxation, stretching, and abdominal muscle-strengthening exercises, I'm going to give you the basic ground rules for doing all of them. *These ground rules are absolutely essential,* and if you do not adhere to them, there is no way you can expect to achieve maximum results. You must follow them. Remember, you have nothing to lose but that crippling back pain. Here are the basic ground rules:

1. Set aside enough time every day to do the Y's Healthy Back exercises. Make that time a holy time for you. Don't do them with the TV or radio on, and if need be, take the phone off the hook. You are *not* to be disturbed. At the Y, we do them in a quiet, darkened room so as not to distract those in the program. Don't do the exercises in the morning shortly after you've gotten out of bed. Your muscles might be too stiff then. Do them later in the day when you've limbered up a bit from normal daily movement.

2. When you begin to do the exercises, do not rush through them. To achieve the maximum benefit, you must take time. It is better not to do the exercises at all if you can't give them enough time. But try to give them the time they require, especially on a

hectic day. That's the day you will need them the most to relieve muscle tension.

3. Do only the exercises that are described in this book, and do not move onto the next exercise before it is called for in the program.

4. As you add new exercises to your weekly program schedule, omit any that cause discomfort. Try them again one week later. If any particular exercise continues to bring discomfort, drop it from your routine entirely.

5. Don't strain by overextending yourself, and avoid jerky movements. Each exercise should be done smoothly.

6. Select a comfortable surface on which to lie. A small mat, such as we use in the Y's program, is highly recommended. Hard floors are taboo.

7. Strip down to your underwear or wear loose fitting attire so that your clothing cannot restrict your movements. Tight clothing is also taboo.

8. If you are currently involved in jogging, running, racquetball, tennis, karate, weight lifting, yoga, fitness classes, or any other physical activity, give it up for now while you are doing the Y's Way to a Healthy Back program. The reason I'm asking you to do this is simple and compelling: the very physical activity you're doing outside the Y's program may be causing your back pain. I can't begin to tell you how many joggers, runners, skiers, tennis players, *et al.* have suffered from back pain induced by their sport. In Chapter 10, I'll show you how you can integrate your activity with the Y's program so you can avoid future episodes of back pain. This program will not only help you in that regard, it will also greatly assist in improving your performance when you return to sports. So don't concern yourself that you'll be missing out for six weeks, because you're going to be ahead of the game when you resume your sports activity.

Now that you know the ground rules, you're ready to begin the Y's Way to a Healthy Back program, by far the most effective of its kind in the world.

CHAPTER
4
The First Week

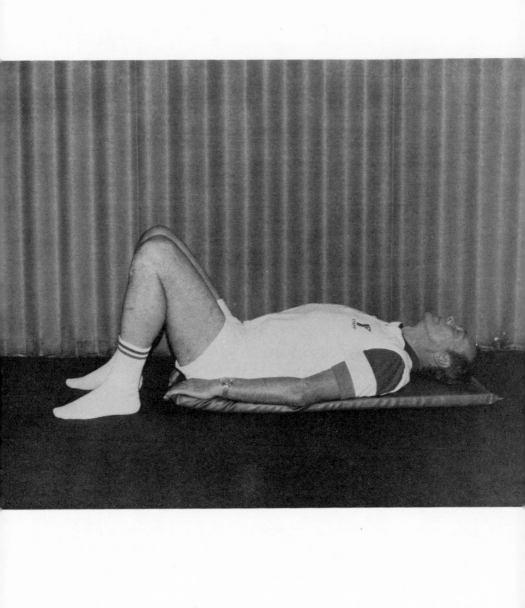

The exercises you are about to do are very easy. They are so easy you might doubt that they will be of help to you in preventing, reducing or eliminating back pain. Cast any such doubt out of your mind. Our statistical records show that 4 out of 5 people who complete the Y's Way to a Healthy Back program attain relief, if not outright elimination of pain.

To start, do *only* the exercises given in this chapter for the first week. If you feel extra spry as a result, don't jump ahead and try to "better" yourself by doing exercises given in the chapter for the second week. You could do yourself harm. If these exercises seem too easy, don't cut back on them. Do what you're supposed to do, no more and no less, according to the program.

When you exercise by yourself, there is a temptation to rush, to get the exercises "out of the way." Don't hurry to get through them. It is important that you take your time, but don't dilly-dally either. As a rule of thumb, allow two or three seconds between each exercise movement. In total, the exercise program for this first week should take you only about 12–15 minutes each day. Remember, you must do the exercises every day to achieve maximum results. If you fail to carry through on that basis, you're only cheating yourself, and your problem is very likely to persist. To get the most out of the exercises, choose a location that is removed from noise and any other distractions that might inter-

LIBRARY
ATLANTIC CHRISTIAN COLLEGE
WILSON. N. C.
87- 2371

fere with your concentration while you are doing them. Finally, if any particular exercise is uncomfortable to perform, do not do it.

When you are ready to start exercising, remove your shoes, leave your socks on, and strip down to your underclothes or wear comfortable clothing. Lie down on your back on a firm mattress or an exercise mat. Don't exercise on a soft mattress or a hard floor because you can hurt yourself.

You are now ready to begin the Y's program. But, before you can actually begin you need to assume what is called "The Basic Position." This means that you must be lying flat on your back with both knees bent and arms at your sides as shown here. The basic position is used as a starting point in many of the exercises throughout the program.

The First Day of the First Week

Exercise 1. This exercise is divided into three parts, A, B, and C.

Exercise 1A. Leg Slide.

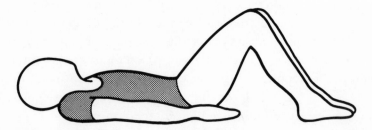

Exercise 1A. Lie flat on your back and close your eyes. Remove all non-exercise thoughts from your mind. Concentrate on the exercise you are about to do. This helps you achieve a more relaxed state of mind, which in turn helps immensely to release tension in your muscles.

Assume the basic position with your arms at your sides, bend your knees as shown. Take a deep breath and exhale slowly through your mouth. Now slide one leg forward on the mat so that the leg is fully extended and resting on the mat. Slide the leg back to the bent knee position. Now do the same exercise with the other leg. Take another deep breath. Exhale slowly. After you have done that, clench both fists and then let them go (loose).

Exercise 1B. Arm Exercise.

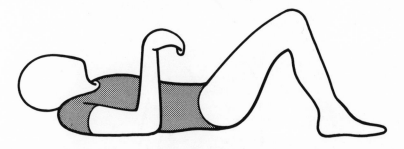

Exercise 1B. Bend one arm *at the elbow* and let it drop easily to the mat. Do the same exercise with the other arm. Take a deep breath and exhale slowly through your mouth.

Exercise 1C. Leg Slide.

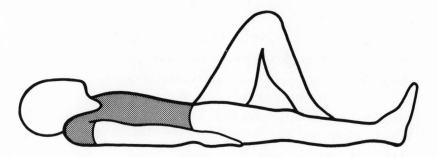

Exercise 1C. This is almost the same exercise as 1A. Slide one leg forward on the mat so that the leg is fully extended and resting on the mat. Slide the leg back to the bent knee position. Now do the same exercise with the other leg. After you have done that, stretch out the fingers of both hands and let them relax.

Exercise 2. Shoulder Shrug.

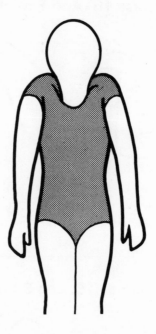

Exercise 2. Take a deep breath and exhale slowly through your mouth. Shrug your shoulders and let them go loose. To do this exercise correctly, slide your shoulders up toward your ears along the mat. Do not lift your shoulders off the mat. If you raise your shoulders off the mat, you will cause tension in the shoulders which defeats the purpose of the exercise. Do this exercise twice more.

Exercise 3. Head Roll.

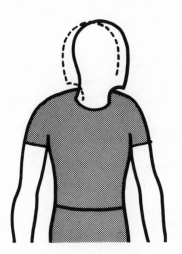

Exercise 3. Take a deep breath and exhale slowly through your mouth. Now let your head fall to one side. Slowly roll your head to the opposite side. I repeat, do this slowly. Be sure you do not force your head to turn more than its natural weight will permit. This exercise helps to reduce tension and stiffness in the neck muscles. One man I know who took the Y's program says that when he does this exercise he relaxes by imagining that his head is a stone rolling on the bottom of the sea. Do this exercise twice more with your head rolling easily from side to side.

Exercise 4. Alternate Leg Lift.

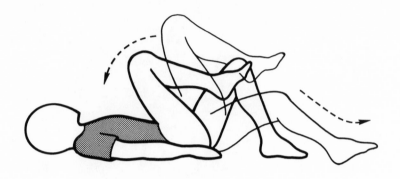

Exercise 4. Take a deep breath and exhale slowly through your mouth. Now bring one knee up toward the shoulder, then return the foot to the mat, sliding the leg all the way out. When the leg is all the way out, slide it back to the starting position. Now bring the other knee up toward the shoulder, return the foot to the mat, and slide the leg all the way out. When the leg is all the way out, slide it back to the starting position. Do this exercise twice more, alternating each leg.

This exercise is designed to release tension and relax the muscles in the middle and lower back. The important thing to keep in mind about this exercise is not to bring the knee too far back. You'll know you're bringing it too far back if you lift your buttock from the mat. If you lift your buttock, you will produce tension, and you want to release tension with the exercise. Just bring the knee up to where it stops naturally without raising the buttock.

Exercise 5. Fetal Position.

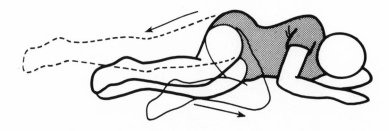

Exercise 5. Turn on either side, eyes closed, so that you assume a "fetal" position, with your head resting comfortably on your underarm. You can place your other arm in front of you or on your hip. Take a deep breath and exhale slowly through your mouth. Remember, keep your eyes closed. Slide the top leg toward your shoulder, letting it fall off the leg beneath it. Now slide the leg out in a straight line as indicated in the illustration, and then slide it back to the starting fetal position. Do this movement twice more.

Roll over onto the other side and assume the fetal position with your eyes closed. Take a deep breath and exhale slowly through your mouth. Do this exercise three times, exactly as you did while lying on the opposite side.

The purpose of this exercise is to relax the muscles in your lower back so as to reduce tension. The important point to bear in mind when you perform this exercise is that the upper leg is always "dead weight" as it slides up toward and then away from the shoulder. The upper leg *always* slides on the under leg. If you lift the leg or raise it even the slightest bit during this exercise, you will produce tension in the low back muscles and defeat the purpose of the exercise.

Exercise 6. Seat Relaxer.

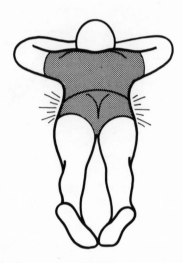

Exercise 6. Roll over onto your stomach with your forehead resting on your folded hands. Point your toes inward. Take a deep breath and exhale slowly through your mouth. Now tighten your buttock muscles. Hold those muscles tight for two seconds and then let go. Do this exercise two more times.

The purpose of this exercise is to release tension in the buttocks area, and pointing your toes inward helps you to isolate your buttock muscles from your leg muscles. Some persons may sense or experience a slight cramping in the soles of the feet. If this happens to you, rotate your feet so they are pointed outward.

Now that you have performed Exercises 1 through 6, repeat them in reverse order, starting with Exercise 5 and ending with Exercise 1.

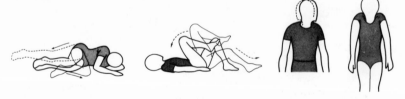

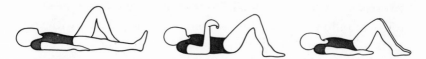

You have now completed your first exercise session. Throughout the six-week program, and later when you continue the exercises on your own, you will always finish the daily program by repeating the exercises in reverse order as we have just done. By doing this, you begin and end with the easiest exercises, and as a result your muscles are relaxed. This is important. Bear it in mind. *Never* build up to a peak and stop there, be it Exercise 6 or 18. Your muscles can become tense that way. You must repeat the exercises in reverse order—back down the scale through Exercise 1.

The Second and Third Day of the First Week

Do exactly the same as the first day. Exercises 1 through 6 and then back down to 1 in reverse order.

The Fourth Day of the First Week

Do Exercises 1 through 6. Now you are ready to add two more exercises to your daily program.

Exercise 7. Double Knee Flex.

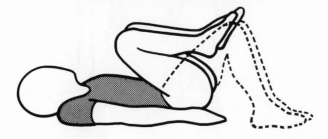

Exercise 7. After doing Exercise 6 while lying on your stomach, roll over onto your back and assume the basic position with your arms at your sides and your knees bent. This new exercise is called the Double Knee Flex. Pull both knees up to your chest, and then gradually lower your legs as you return to your basic starting position with both feet on the floor. Be sure you do not raise your hips off the mat. The Double Knee Flex is designed to start the strengthening of your abdominal muscles. Do the exercise twice more. Next, you add Exercise 8.

Exercise 8. Cat Back.

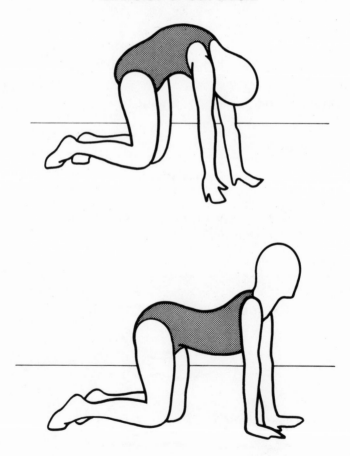

Exercise 8. Assume a kneeling position on all fours so that you are resting on your hands and knees. The exercise you are about to do is called the Cat Back. Arch your back like a cat and at the same time drop your head slowly and tuck in your pelvis. Now reverse the exercise slowly by gently forming a "U" in your back. As you perform this movement, raise your head and stick your buttocks out at the same time. As with all exercises, this one in particular, do it slowly and smoothly. Do it just the way a cat would do it when it gets up from a nap and stretches. Do this exercise twice more. Its purpose is to stretch the back muscles to make them more flexible.

After you have finished doing Exercise 8, do the exercises in reverse order, starting with 7 and ending with 1.

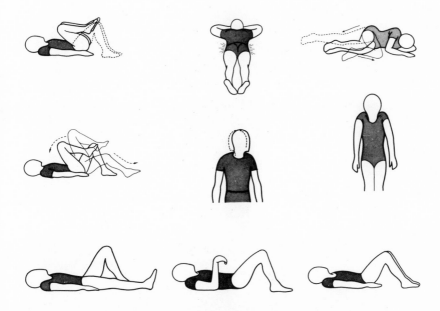

The Fifth, Sixth, and Seventh Day of the First Week

Do exactly the same as the fourth day. Exercises 1 through 8 and then back down through 1 in reverse order.

Again, I cannot stress too much the value to you in being relaxed during the entire course of exercises. It will pay off in helping you eliminate low back pain *and* in reducing the time required to do so.

CHAPTER
5
The Second Week

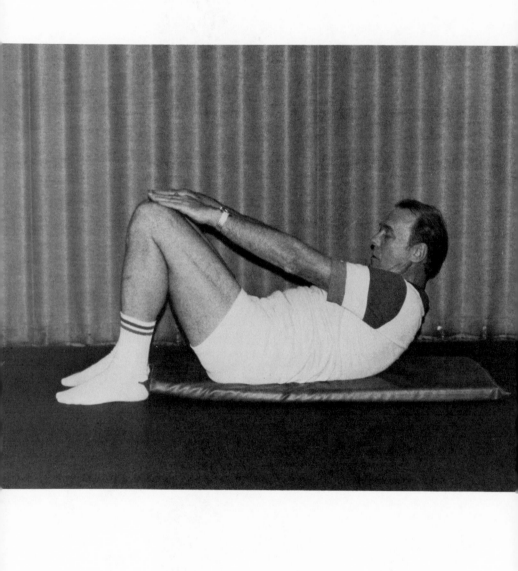

It is usually at this point in the program that I have noticed someone beginning to question the value of the exercises. This is because the exercises seem so easy to do, and some find it hard to believe that such simple movements can really play a role in relieving pain. Accept my word for it. These exercises do help, but you must persist with them daily.

The First Day of the Second Week

Begin this week by doing Exercises 1 through 8 and, as soon as you have completed them, you are ready to add Exercise 9 to your program.

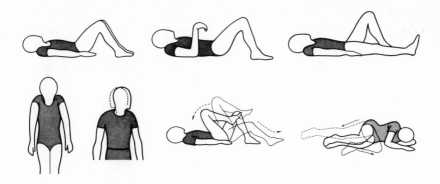

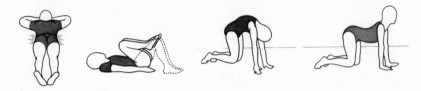

Exercise 9. Half Sit-up.

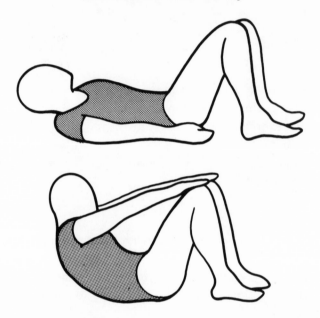

Exercise 9. Assume the basic position on your back, with your arms at your sides and knees bent. Take in a deep breath and exhale slowly through your mouth as you come to a half sit-up position. Bring your fingertips to the tops of your knees. When your fingertips reach your knees, lower your trunk and uncurl slowly until your back, shoulders and head are again resting on the mat. Let all muscles go loose so that you are completely relaxed. Repeat the exercise two more times.

This exercise, which is slightly more demanding than Exercise 7, is designed to increase the strength of the muscles in the abdominal wall.

When you have finished with Exercise 9, reverse the entire order beginning with Exercise 8 and continuing through 7, 6, 5, 4, 3, 2, and 1, doing each three times.

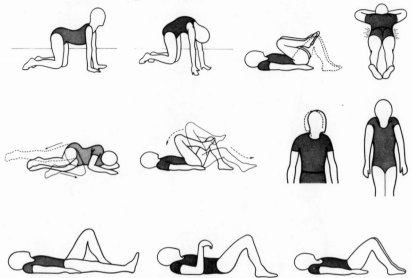

The Second and Third Day of the Second Week

Do exactly the same exercises that you did on the previous day: Exercise 1 through 9 and then back down to 1 in reverse order.

The Fourth Day of the Second Week

Do Exercises 1 through 9. You are now ready to add Exercise 10.

Exercise 10. Pectoral Stretch.

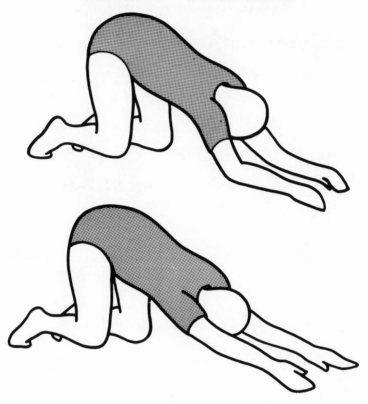

Exercise 10. Turn over to an on-all-fours position. Place your hands, and then your forearms, on the mat. With your thighs at right angles to the mat, slide your forearms forward while you keep your back and head straight. As soon as you begin to feel a pull in the upper chest area, slide your forearms back until you have returned to the "all fours" starting position. Remember to keep your thighs stationary. They remain perpendicular to the mat throughout the entire exercise. Do this exercise two more times.

The Pectoral Stretch is designed to stretch the upper chest muscles, which in turn increases mobility of the shoulders.

After completing Exercise 10, reverse the entire order of exercises by first doing Exercises 9, 8, 7, 6, 5, 4, 3, 2, and 1.

The Fifth, Sixth, and Seventh Day of the Second Week

Do exactly the same exercises that you did the previous day: 1 through 10 and back down to 1 in reverse order.

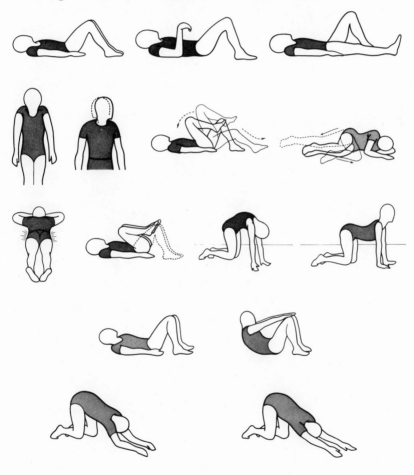

At the end of the second week, about 10% of those in the Y's program begin to feel some relief from pain. For the most part,

their low back pain now appears to have been related to stress and
tension, and they have helped overcome this condition by mas-
tering the relaxation exercises. Typical is the recent case of a
young woman in New York City who enrolled in the Y's Way to a
Healthy Back program. She wrote, "The benefit of the exercises
was clear almost immediately after starting the program. My
back, neck and shoulders were more relaxed. I slept better, and
the tension of one day did not follow me into the next."

CHAPTER
6
The Third Week

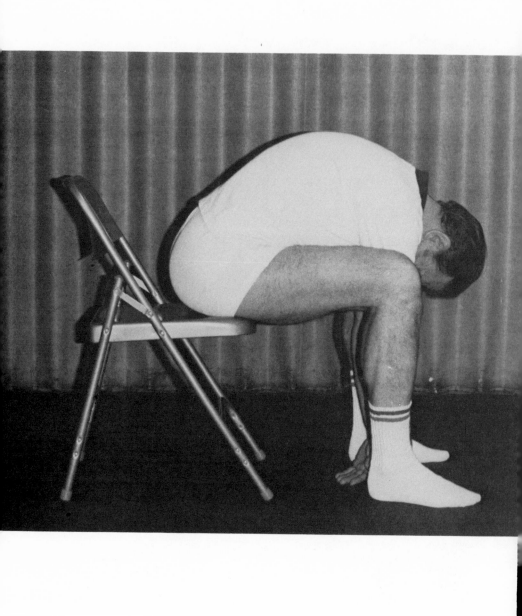

On the first day of this week you will have completed almost one-half of the course. By now you should definitely begin to feel the benefits of the relaxation exercises. Whether you know it or not, your stomach muscles are getting stronger. Again, numerous advances and benefits in the elimination of low back pain and muscle weakness will have taken place almost without your noticing them. These are important elements in the overall Healthy Back program, and because of them you are well on your way to having a healthy back again. Keep up the good work.

The First Day of the Third Week

Do Exercises 1 through 10. You are now ready to add Exercise 11.

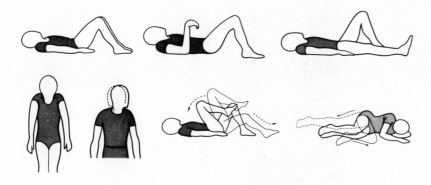

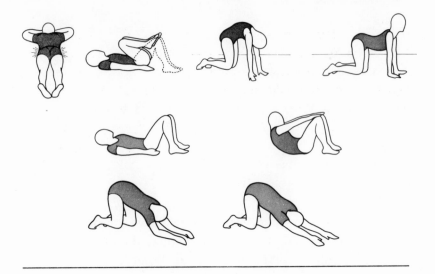

Exercise 11. Bend Sitting.

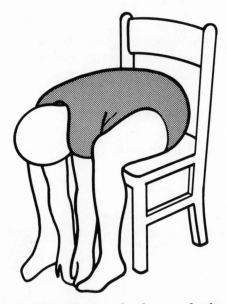

Exercise 11. You will need a sturdy chair to do this exercise. Sit forward in the chair so that part of your body weight is borne by your feet and legs. This helps stabilize your position in the chair.

Spread your legs so that your head and arms will be able to pass through them. Now, slowly bend toward the floor by letting your chin drop on your chest and allowing your shoulders to sag. Let your shoulders come down between your knees, arms dangling. Hang loose, as the saying goes, for about five seconds. Now return smoothly and easily to a straight sitting position and relax. Do this exercise two more times.

This bend exercise stretches the back muscles. Be sure that you don't jerk, bounce or force yourself downward.

When you have finished Exercise 11, reverse the entire order, starting with Exercises 10 and 9.

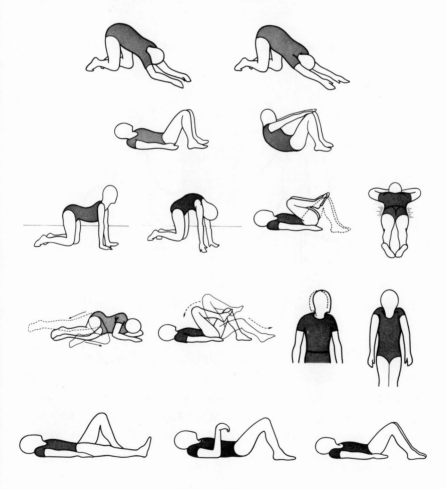

The Second and Third Day of the Third Week

Do exactly the same exercises as you did the previous day, Exercises 1 through 11 and back down to 1 in reverse order.

The Fourth Day of the Third Week

Do exercises 1 through 11. You are now ready to add Exercise 12.

Exercise 12. Sit-up with Feet Secured.

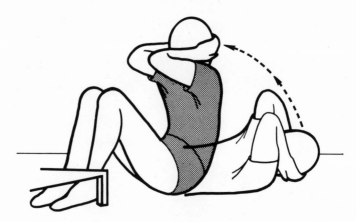

Exercise 12. You will need to have someone or something hold your feet down when you do this exercise. If you are alone, use a heavy object, such as a bureau or a couch, that won't topple. With your back on the mat, and your feet held down firmly, bring your buttocks as close to your heels as feels comfortable and without placing undue strain on your knees. Place your hands at the sides of your head and take a deep breath. Exhale slowly through your mouth and slowly curl up into a sitting position. Now lower yourself back to the mat by uncurling to the starting position.

When your back is again on the mat, relax your shoulders. Do this exercise two more times.

Don't try to do this exercise by jerking yourself forward or holding your trunk stiff. That defeats the purpose. If you find that you can't do the full sit-up, do not be discouraged. Your abdominal muscles need strengthening, which will come in time, and you should go about it gradually. Instead of placing your hands at the sides of your head, put them at your sides on the mat when you try the sit-up. When your abdominal muscles get stronger, cross your hands over your stomach. When your abdominal muscles gain even more strength, do the sit-up with your arms crossed on your chest. Finally, do the sit-up with your hands placed at the sides of your head.

Many people in the Healthy Back program are unable to do a full sit-up even with their arms at their sides. This is not surprising. After all, the sit-up is one of the Kraus–Weber Tests. If you can't even do the sit-up with your arms at your sides, stay with the earlier exercises until your abdominal muscles have gained enough strength for you to do the sit-up that way. Then move on with the day-by-day program. Most students who fail to do a full-fledged sit-up at first are able to do one by the end of six weeks, and for many of them this is the first time they have been able to do one in years.

After you have done Exercise 12, you go back down in reverse order starting with Exercise 11 and ending with 1. If I seem repetitive in saying this, it's because I mean to be. In each Healthy Back class I teach, I am always reminding and coaching the correct procedures.

The Fifth, Sixth, and Seventh Day of the Third Week

Do Exercises 1 through 12, then do them back down to 1 in descending reverse order.

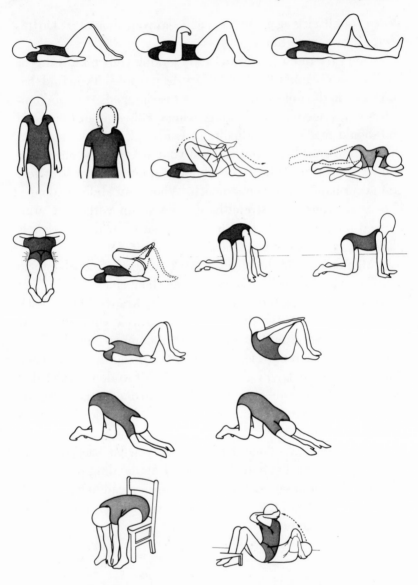

By the end of the third week, 15 to 20 percent of those enrolled in the Y's program have experienced reduced pain. Again, loss of muscular stress and tension appears to be the reason, along with an increase of strength of the abdominal muscles.

CHAPTER

7

The Fourth Week

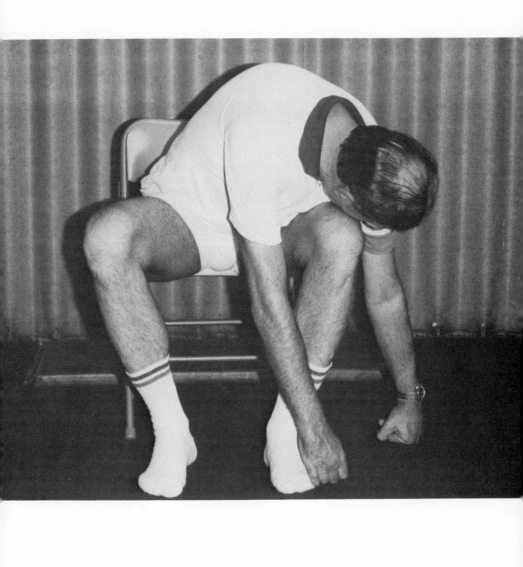

You have now completed one-half of the six week program. Well done! Again, I urge you not to be misled by the simplicity and ease with which you can do the exercises. Benefits for the majority who religiously follow the program will begin to be apparent from this point onward.

The First Day of the Fourth Week

Do Exercises 1 through 12. You are now ready to do Exercise 13.

Exercise 13. Bend Sitting Rotation.

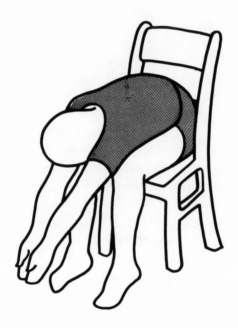

Exercise 13. As with Exercise 11, you will need a sturdy chair. Sit forward in the chair so that part of your body weight is borne by the feet and legs. But this time, spread your legs only slightly. With both arms resting at your sides, bring them forward and down to the right side, as illustrated. When you have come down as far as you can without forcing—hang loose for about 5 seconds.

Now come up slowly, sliding your arms across your thighs to the other side. Pause briefly, and bend down slowly toward the floor and hang loose for 5 seconds. Do this exercise two more times to each side. Always hang loose. Don't strain or use bouncy or jerky movements.

The purpose of this exercise is to further increase the flexibility and stretchability of your back muscles.

Now do the exercises in reverse: 12, 11, 10, 9, 8, 7, 6, 5, 4, 3, 2, and 1.

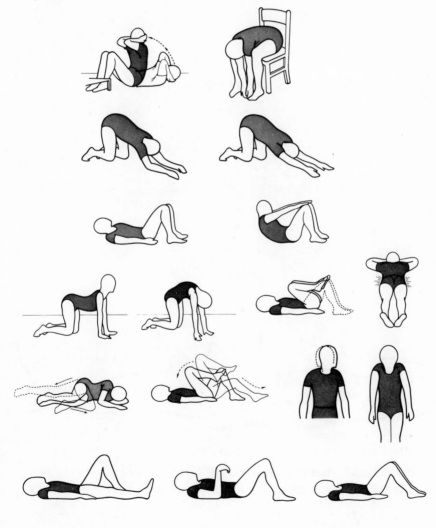

The Second and Third Day of the Fourth Week

Do exactly the same exercises that you did the previous day: Exercises 1 through 13 and then back down to 1 in reverse order.

The Fourth Day of the Fourth Week

Do Exercises 1 through 13. You are now ready to add Exercise 14.

Exercise 14. First Hamstring Stretch.

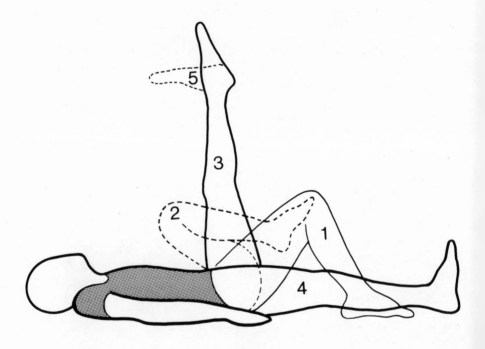

Exercise 14. Assume the basic position on your back on the mat (1), with your arms at your sides and your knees bent. The

numbers on the illustration of this exercise and in the description correspond to the various movements.

Bring one knee up toward your chest (2), then extend the leg in a straight line toward the ceiling and "lock" it in this position by locking the knee. As you extend the straight leg toward the ceiling, also point your toes toward the ceiling (3). When the leg is fully extended, keep it straight and lower it to the mat without bending it. As the straight leg comes to rest on the mat (4), slide it back to the starting bent-knee position (1) and relax.

Repeat this movement with the other leg.

When you have completed this movement once with each leg you are to change the exercise slightly. This time start with the right leg, but as you extend it in a straight line toward the ceiling, "cup" the heel by pointing your toes toward your head (5). Be sure to keep the leg locked in a straight line as you do so. Now lower the straight leg to the mat, rest it briefly, and slide it back to the starting bent-knee position.

Do the same with the left leg. Repeat this exercise once more with each leg, alternately pointing the toes straight and cupping the heel.

The purpose of this exercise is to stretch the muscles at the back of the thighs and calf muscles of the leg.

When you have completed Exercise 14, reverse the order by doing 13, 12, 11, 10, 9, 8, 7, 6, 5, 4, 3, 2, and 1.

The Fifth, Sixth, and Seventh Day of the Fourth Week

Do exactly the same exercises that you did the previous day: Exercises 1 through 14, and then back down to 1 in descending reverse order.

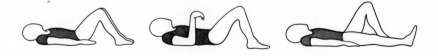

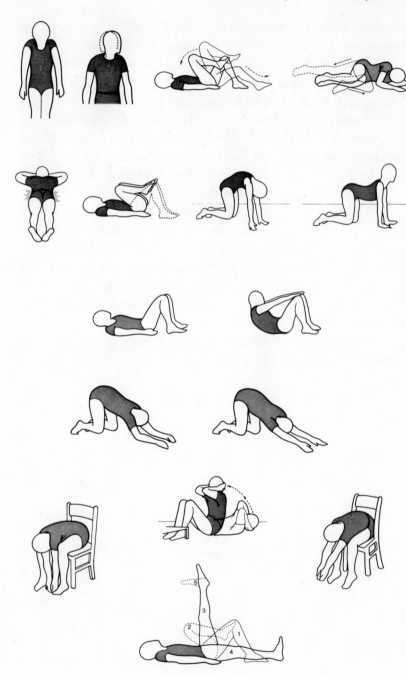

Our experience with the Y's Way to a Healthy Back program shows that at this point about half those in the program have begun to find real relief from pain. If you have, good for you. Your muscles have been tense and stiff, but at long last you are learning how to relax through exercise. If you have not felt any relief from pain, please do not be discouraged. Remember, this is a six-week course. You are already two-thirds of the way there and for most the benefits can be expected to become progressively greater.

CHAPTER
8
The Fifth Week

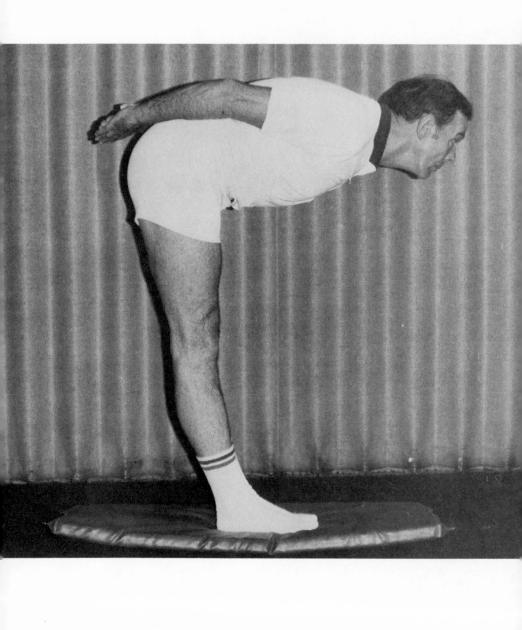

The First Day of the Fifth Week

You will notice by now that your persistence in doing the relaxing exercises daily is beginning to pay off for you. This week and next you'll add a series of stretching exercises designed to improve muscle flexibility. Not only will you become more flexible, you will notice that you are able to handle your body weight more easily.

Begin your session today by doing Exercises 1 through 14. You are now ready to add Exercise 15.

Exercise 15. Second Hamstring Stretch.

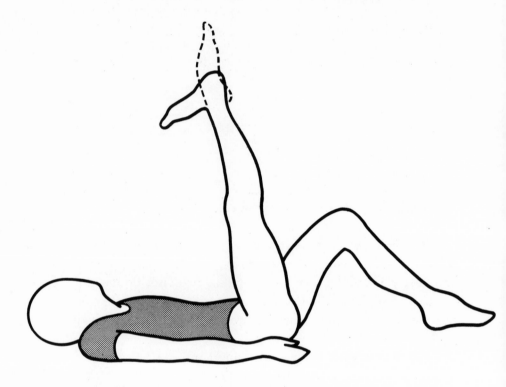

Exercise 15. Assume the basic position on your back on the mat with your arms at your sides and your knees bent.

Slide the right leg forward on the mat, pointing your toes away from you. With the knee locked, slowly raise the straightened leg as high as you can, with toes also pointed straight. Make sure you do not bend your knee. Lower the leg, still straight, to the mat, slide it back up to the starting position, and relax.

Do the same movement with the left leg.

Do the same with the right leg again, but this time point your toes toward your head so that your heel is pointing up.

Do the same exercise with the left leg. Repeat this exercise once with each leg.

When doing this exercise, do not raise your leg quickly or kick it upward. Make sure not to bend your knee. If you bend the knee, you will negate the purpose of this stretching exercise.

After you do Exercise 15, do Exercises 14, 13, 12, 11, 10, and 9, and 8, 7, 6, 5, 4, 3, 2, and 1 in reverse order.

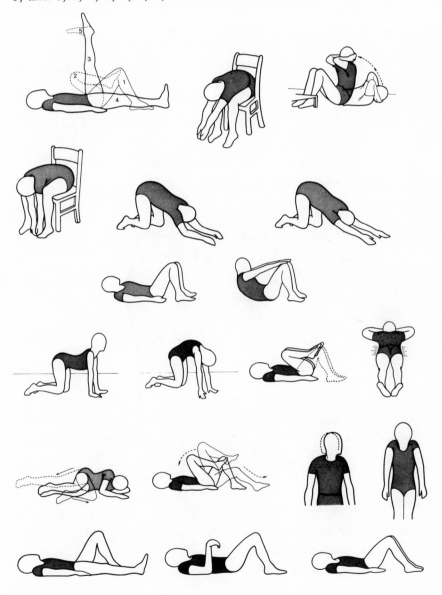

The Second and Third Day of the Fifth Week

Do exactly the same exercises that you did the previous day: Exercises 1 through 15 and back down to 1 in reverse order.

The Fourth Day of the Fifth Week

Do Exercises 1 through 15. You are now ready to add Exercise 16.

Exercise 16. Hamstring Stretch, Standing.

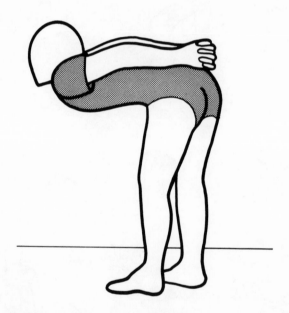

Exercise 16. Stand up and spread your legs apart to approximately the width of your shoulders. Put your arms behind your back and clasp your hands. Rest your arms on your back and keep them straight by locking them at the elbows.

Slowly bend forward from the waist keeping your head up. Bend forward as far as you can until you feel stretching in the backs of your knees. When you do, hold this position for two seconds and straighten up. This exercise lengthens the muscles in the backs of your legs.

When you do this exercise, do not strain or jerk forward.

Do this exercise two more times. After you do Exercise 16, do the exercises in reverse order, 15, 14, 13, 12, 11, 10, and 9, and 8, 7, 6, 5, 4, 3, 2, and 1.

The Fifth, Sixth, and Seventh Day of the Fifth Week

Do exactly the same exercises that you did the previous day: Exercises 1 through 16 and then back down to 1 in reverse order.

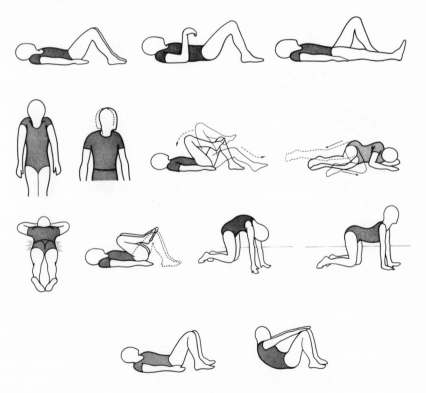

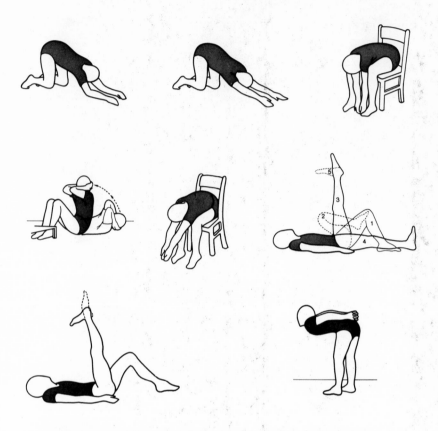

After the fifth week, 60–65 percent of those in the Y's program feel less back pain. Muscle toning and stretching have begun to play a very significant role in relieving low back pain.

CHAPTER
9
The Sixth and Final Week

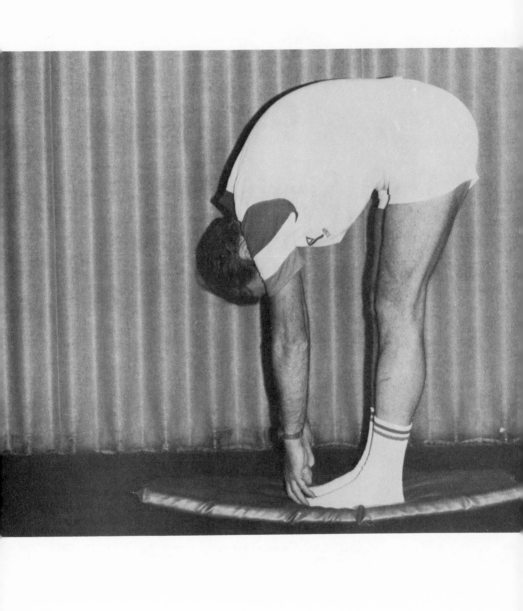

The First Day of the Sixth and Final Week

There is no doubt that most of you who have regularly followed the exercise plan will now have less back pain. As you begin the sixth and final week of the program, just because you have not noticed an appreciable lessening of pain, don't be discouraged. It just takes some people a bit longer to gain the benefits of the program. I urge you to stay with it; don't quit.

First, do Exercises 1 through 16. You are now ready to add Exercise 17.

Exercise 17. Calf Muscle Stretch.

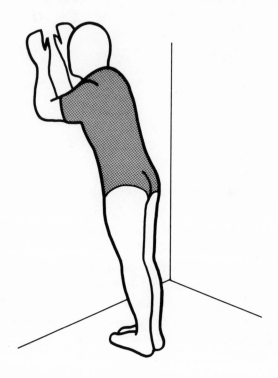

Exercise 17. Take a standing position in front of a wall. Stand away from the wall a little more than arm's length, feet together, and back and hips straight. Place your hands flat on the wall opposite your shoulders. Lean toward the wall, bending your arms at the elbow, until your forearms come in contact with it. Then use your arms to push your body back to the standing position. Relax.

Make sure to keep your body straight. Do not bend at the waist, and keep your heels in contact with the floor at all times.

Do this exercise two more times. It is excellent for stretching your calf muscles.

Now do the exercises in reverse, 16, 15, 14, 13, 12, 11, 10, 9, 8, 7, 6, 5, 4, 3, 2, and 1, followed by Exercise 18, the last in the Healthy Back program.

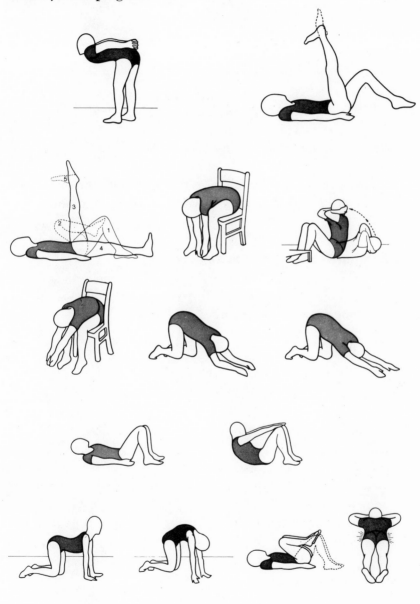

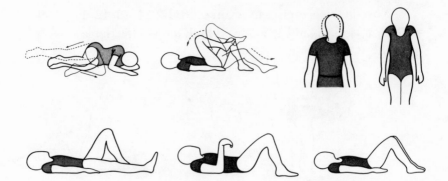

The Second and Third Day of the Sixth Week

Do exactly the same exercises that you did the previous day, 1 through 17, and then back down to 1 in reverse order.

The Fourth Day of the Sixth Week

Do Exercises 1 through 17. You are now ready to add the final exercise in the program.

Exercise 18. Floor Touch (Floor Reach).

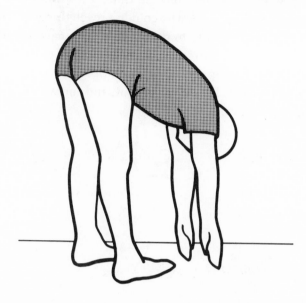

Exercise 18. This is the peak exercise in the program. First you must warm-up. Stand up straight, and spread your legs about the width of your shoulders. Now relax by inhaling deeply and exhaling slowly through your mouth. Keeping your knees locked, lower your head gradually and let your trunk hang loose from the hips. Drop your shoulders and then your back gradually as your arms and hands hang down toward the floor. Let gravity help you. Don't strain. Now straighten up. Do this warm-up movement two or three times until you feel completely relaxed. Once you're relaxed, repeat the exercise, but this time reach for the floor with your fingertips. Reach as far down as you comfortably can without straining. Now straighten up to a standing position. Do the exercise twice. If your fingertips touch the floor, you have finished the Y's Way to a Healthy Back program right on schedule. At this point, eighty percent of those who have completed the program will have experienced relief or complete elimination of low back pain. Whether or not you are able to touch

the floor with your fingertips, you will continue to do the full
exercise program—exercises 1 through 18 and then back down to
1 in reverse order—every day. In time, a few weeks, perhaps a
few months, most of those who couldn't reach the floor with their
fingertips should be able to do so. Once you have been able to
touch the floor, do this exercise with your legs together. But even
if you can't do it, keep on with the full program on a daily basis.
Your muscles need a full daily workout, and you will be the better
for it in many ways.

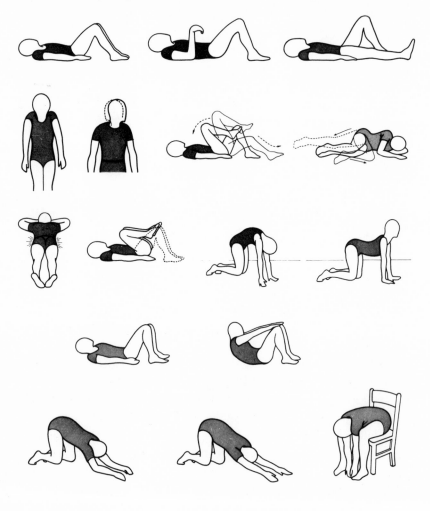

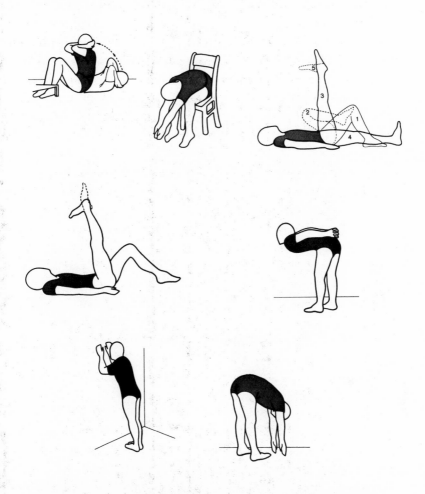

I recall the case of a friend, Jack O., who took the Y's program after he had hurt his back as the result of an automobile accident.

He let two years go by before he embarked on the exercise program you've just learned here. I say "learned" and not "finished" because you're never finished with this program, which is the point of my story about Jack. By the end of six weeks, Jack couldn't touch the floor. The best he could do was to get within five inches of it. I was not in the least surprised because when Jack started the program he could barely touch his knees. I told him he had to continue with the program on his own. He did, and it took him another four months before he could finally touch the floor. He kept up with the program for another several months, but then, as he admitted to me later, he began to slack off, especially when he had a "busy day." Jack was and is a tense man to begin with, and after a number of busy days went by and he failed to exercise, his muscles began to tense and stiffen, especially his hamstrings. When he did do the exercises he did them only sporadically, and because he was incapable of doing the full set he began cutting back more and more. Finally, he stopped entirely. About four months later, he felt a sharp pull in his lower back while he was splitting wood with a maul. He gave the log another whack, and this time there was a sharper pull and sharp pain. Jack's back was out of whack. He hobbled into bed, gave me a call and "fessed" up. "Jack," I told him, "you have only yourself to blame. I'm not going to come down on you hard and say that I warned you, but I did tell you that you had to continue with the full program every day. There is absolutely no point in your taking the program again at the Y because you've been through it here and you know it. When your back pain eases off in a couple of days, just start doing the program again at home as if you were a complete newcomer. Do Exercise 1 through 6 for the first four days, then start adding on just as you did in the program. Don't try to jump ahead and do the full set in three weeks. You need to take your time, and once you have returned to doing the full program, keep it up *every* day, or the same thing is going to happen to you again. And be especially sure to do the exercises, the full program, on those days when you have been unusually busy, because that's when you'll need the exercises the most in order to get rid of the day's tensions that have accumulated in your muscles."

Jack said he would, and he did. He's all right now. Let his case be a lesson. Continue to do the exercises every day. The only times you'll make an exception to this is on days when you play sports or engage in other vigorous exercises. If you do that, you can modify the program by doing selective exercises. I'll show you how to do just that in Chapter 10.

CHAPTER

10

The Sports Follow-Up Program

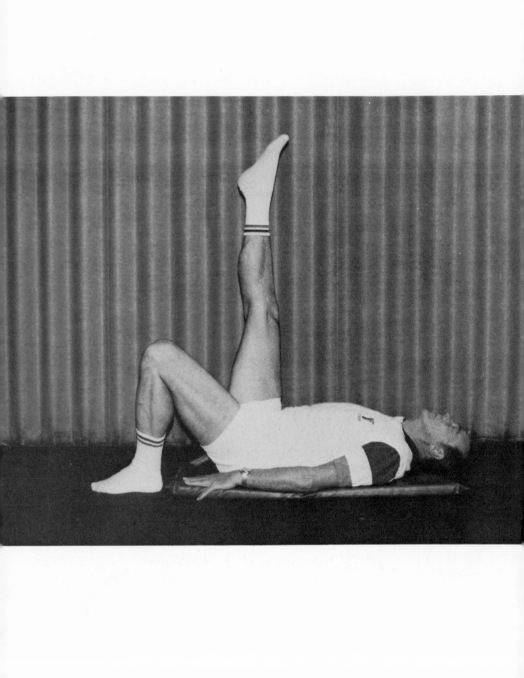

Now that you have completed the six-week program, you may want to resume sports or vigorous other physical activities. By all means do so. Earlier I advised you to stop while you were learning the Y's exercises because our experience shows that maximum results are achieved when participants confine themselves to the Y's exercises alone during the six-week period. Once you're ready to resume sports, you'll find that you haven't lost your edge at all. In fact, you will have gained an advantage because your muscles are now stronger and more flexible, and that will help to offset injury. Marty Snelling, physical director of the Toronto YMCA, has a marathon club with several hundred members. Sixty to seventy of them will run in a given race, but before the marathon begins, they all do the relaxing and stretching exercises from the Healthy Back program. After finishing the race, each runner exercises again. Marty estimates that as a result the club has cut injuries by 75 percent.

I wish I could impress the value of exercise on every athletic coach in the country. There are certain sports in which it is impossible to prevent injury because of the very nature of the game, such as football (and I include touch football). But in most sports it is possible to limit physical injuries and it is tragic that so many coaches are unaware of the benefits of the exercises to athletes. I have a friend who is a sportswriter, and after he read Hans Kraus' book, *Sports Injuries*, he said to me, "Al, if I were a millionaire and owned a professional team, I believe the team would be in the World Series, the NBA finals, or even the Super Bowl within the space of two years, no matter how bad it was when I bought it. And I'll tell you how I'd do it. I'd get every athlete who had been injured and released by his club, and I'd have Dr. Kraus or someone else truly expert in the field of physical medicine and rehabilitation examine them one by one. Dr. Kraus might say, 'Forget this one. His knees are shot,' but then he might say, 'This pitcher has a triggerpoint in his shoulder. After treatment he should be fine.' And so on. I'd take all these reconditioned athletes and put together a team that would beat everyone in sight. And it would be so easy to do because so many people in sports haven't the slightest idea of what correct exercise can do."

Keep my sportswriter friend's enthusiasm and insights in mind when you participate in sports. The right exercises can do so much for you. This may sound contradictory, but the best thing that happened to a marathon runner I know was that he injured his back. He hadn't been warming up properly, but after he went on an exercise program to correct his condition he resumed his running and he did better than ever before because the exercises had lengthened his stride and he could eat up the ground.

I am by no means suggesting that you're going to win the Boston Marathon or the country club singles tennis tournament simply because you exercise regularly, but I do believe you are going to perform at the peak of your personal abilities if you do. Here is what you should do. On the days that you do not run or play sports or do "your thing," do all the Healthy Back exercises, 1 to 18, and then back down to 1 in reverse order. Remember, you do *each* exercise three times. But, and this is important, on the days when you do participate in your sport, you will modify the Healthy Back program. You do the exercises in two sessions, one before and one after. The first exercise session is designed to warm you up. It is absolutely essential that you warm up properly before you go out on the court, on the track or wherever. A proper warm-up will prepare your muscles for strenuous activity so that sudden or repetitive movements will not cause you to suffer muscle strain or injury.

Here is the warm-up as modified from the regular exercise program. Again, do Exercises 1 through 6, all three times each.

Exercise 1A. Leg Slide.

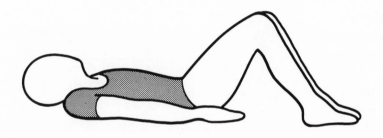

Exercise 1B. Arm Exercise.

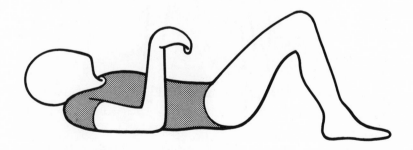

Exercise 1C. Leg Slide.

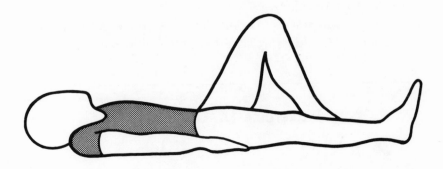

Exercise 2. Shoulder Shrug.

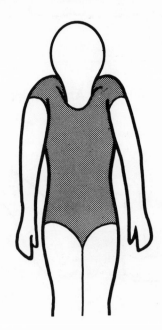

Exercise 3. Head Roll.

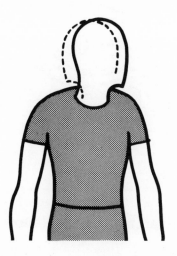

Exercise 4. Alternate Leg Lift.

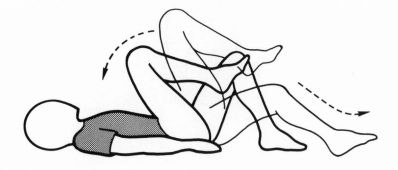

Exercise 5. Fetal Position.

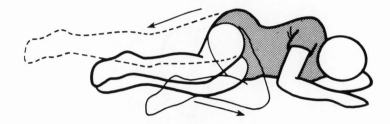

Exercise 6. Seat Relaxer.

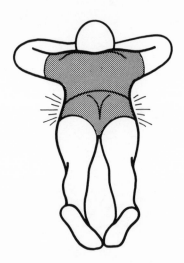

After completing Exercise 6, do Exercise 8, illustrated again for convenience.

Exercise 8. Cat Back.

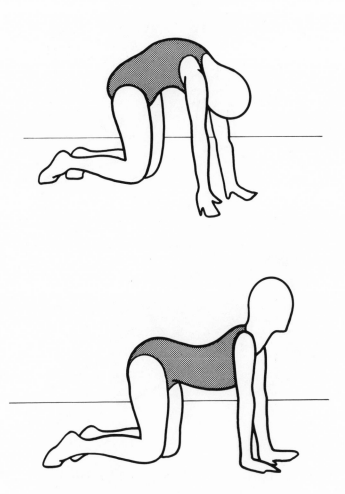

After you do Exercise 8, do Exercise 10.

Exercise 10. Pectoral Stretch.

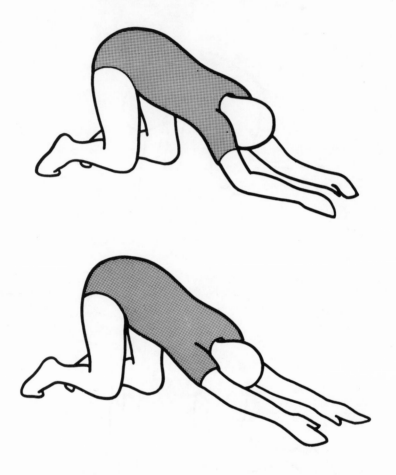

When you have completed Exercise 10, jump ahead to Exercise 14.

Exercise 14. The First Hamstring Stretch.

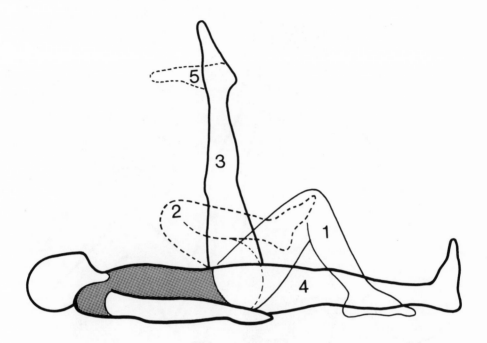

After doing Exercise 14, move on to 15.

Exercise 15. The Second Hamstring Stretch.

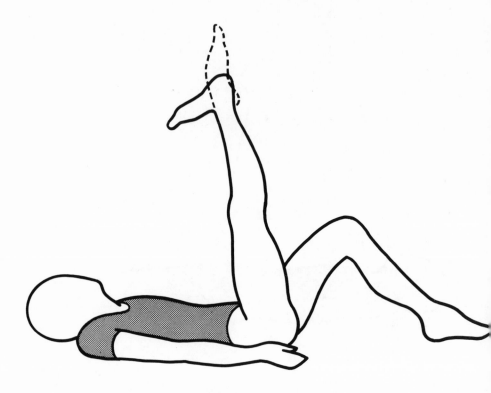

Next do Exercise 16.

Exercise 16. Hamstring Stretch, Standing.

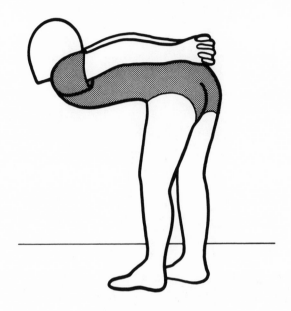

Following Exercise 16, do Exercise 17.

Exercise 17. Calf Muscle Stretch.

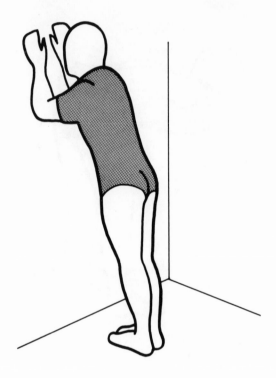

Finally, as part of the proper warm-up, do Exercise 18.

Exercise 18. Floor Touch (Floor Reach).

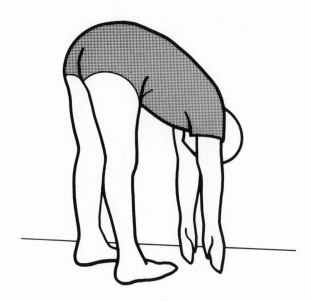

Now that you have done these exercises for your warm-up, you are ready to take part in vigorous physical activity. A couple of points to bear in mind. If you're a runner or a jogger, don't believe that jogging or running is a warm-up in itself. It is not. If you don't do the above exercises beforehand, you can injure yourself. You must prepare your body for jogging or running.

Long-distance joggers and runners covering five miles or more in a workout should add the following exercises to their warm-up routine.

Exercise 19. Runner's Calf Stretch.

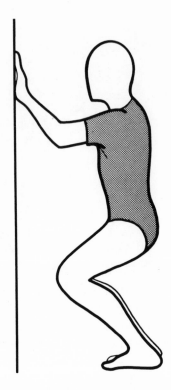

Exercise 19. Move to a standing position in front of a wall. Stand back from the wall approximately 6 inches more than an arm's length. With your body straight and feet together, lean into the wall with your hands flat on the wall opposite your shoulders. From this position you now move into a squat position, keeping your heels in contact with the floor. After you have gone down as far as you can, without straining, come up to a standing position, still keeping your hands in contact with the wall. Do this exercise two more times. It stretches the soleus muscle and minimizes injury to the Achilles area.

Exercise 20. Sitting Stretch.

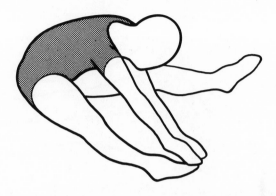

Exercise 20. Sit with legs flat on the mat and spread apart. Point the toes away from you comfortably. Slowly bend forward and touch the toes of your right foot with the fingers of both hands. Return to the upright position. Repeat this movement twice. Now do the same exercise with the left foot. Return to the upright position. Repeat this movement twice.

Exercise 21. Hurdle Sit.

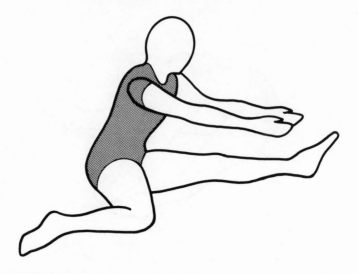

Exercise 21. Sit with your left leg flat on the mat, straight out, toes pointed away from you comfortably. The right leg is bent behind you easily, as if you were hurdling a fence. Do not strain. Slowly bend forward and touch the toes of the left foot with the fingertips of both hands. Return to the upright position. Repeat this movement twice.

Now bring the right leg to the straight-out, flat position, toes forward easily. Place the left leg behind you in the hurdling position. Slowly bend forward and touch the toes of the right foot with the fingertips of both hands. Return to the upright position. Repeat this movement twice.

Exercise 22. Quadriceps Stretch.

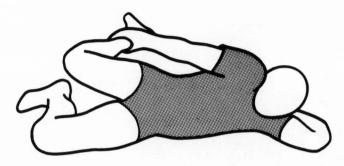

Exercise 22. Lie on your left side with legs bent behind you, left arm beneath the head for support. Grasp the right ankle and pull the leg back slowly toward the buttocks as far as you comfortably can, stretching the front thigh muscle. Repeat two more times. Then roll over on your right side and repeat three times with your left leg.

In his book, *Sports Injuries,* Dr. Hans Kraus advises that anyone participating in a sport involving strenuous use of the legs add the following warm-up exercise. Do it after completing those listed above.

Exercise 23. Flutter Kick.

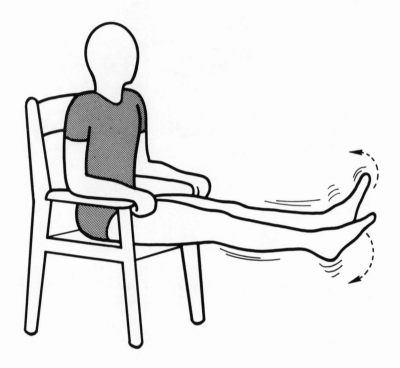

Exercise 23. Sit on the edge of a chair, legs straight out, and alternately kick each one rapidly 50 to 100 times as though you were swimming.

If you are about to engage in vigorous physical activity that involves the arms and shoulders as well, such as tennis, also add the following warm-up.

Exercise 24. Full Arm Circle Swing.

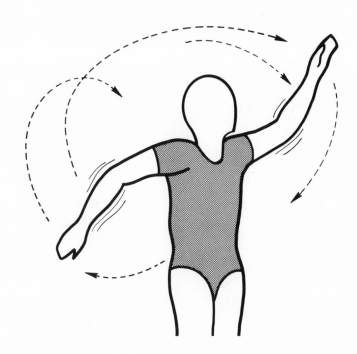

Exercise 24. Standing, swing your arms backward and forward, up and down, rapidly 50 to 100 times as though you were trying to warm yourself on a cold day.

After you have finished your sport activity, you must cool off properly. Your muscles need to relax. Here is what you should do.

Walk slowly until your heart rate drops to 100 beats or less per minute. When it has dropped to that level, do Exercises 1 through 6. After you finish Exercise 6, go to Exercise 14, as illustrated.

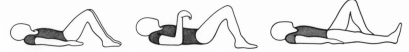

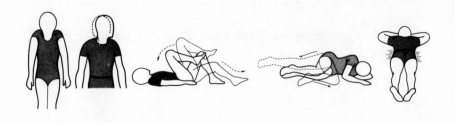

Exercise 14. First Hamstring Stretch, Knee Bent.

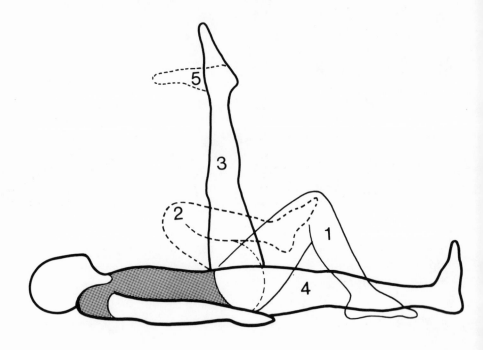

After doing Exercise 14, do Exercise 15.

Exercise 15. Second Hamstring Stretch, Knee Locked.

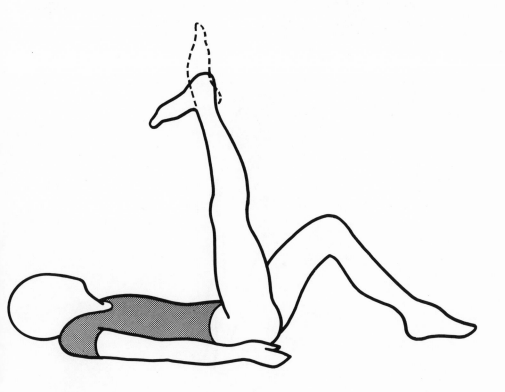

Then do Exercise 17.

Exercise 17. Calf Muscle Stretch.

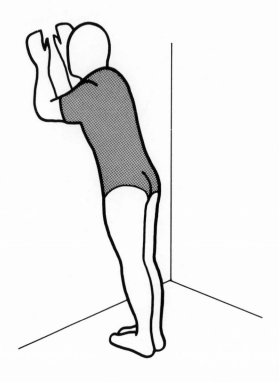

Next, do Exercise 18.

Exercise 18. Floor Touch (Floor Reach).

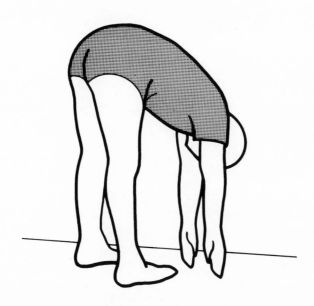

When you finish Exercise 18, you go back down the exercises given in this chapter in reverse order to Exercise 10.

After finishing Exercise 10, jump down to Exercise 8.

When you have finished Exercise 8, do Exercises 6 through 1 in that order to complete your cool-off session. The warm-up and cool-off sessions constitute your full exercise program on days when you indulge in sports or vigorous physical activity. Remember, on days that you don't, you must do Exercises 1 through 18 and then back down to 1 in reverse order.

CHAPTER

11

The Walk to
Health Program

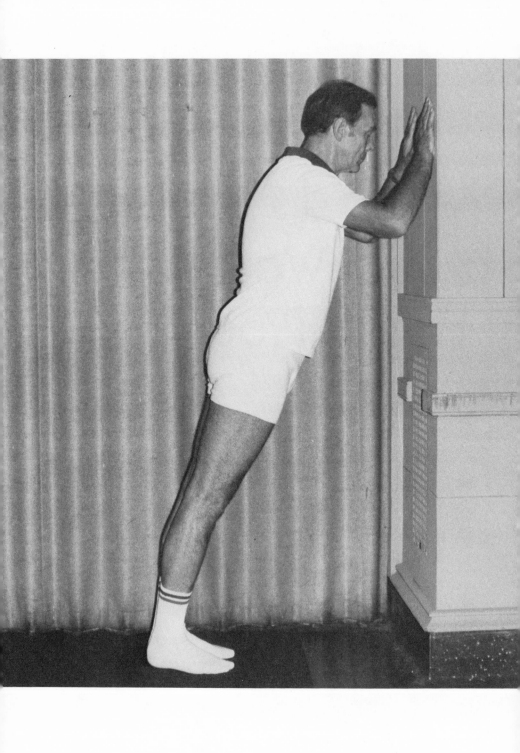

If you're not active in sports, one of the best things you can do for your body and peace of mind is to walk. Yes, walk. As Dr. George Sheehan, the famous marathon-running cardiologist, says, "I think jogging is completely unnecessary for a fitness program. A good, long, brisk walk is equivalent to a jog anytime."

There have been many famous walkers throughout history who considered this natural activity essential. Some of the more recent well-known walkers were former President Harry Truman and Albert Einstein. Abraham Lincoln and Thomas Jefferson were walkers, as was William Wordsworth. Bob Hope is a walker. He took up walking years ago when he was on the road doing vaudeville. Even now, after doing a TV show or making a public appearance, Hope regularly will walk two to four miles.

There are many advantages to a walking program. Charles Kuntzleman, Ed.D., one of our country's leading authorities on this activity, tested the concepts of walking with groups in the communities of Jackson and Grand Rapids, Michigan, and Allentown, Pennsylvania. The results were astonishing. Not only did the walkers lose weight and body fat, they also lowered their blood pressures and cholesterol levels in the blood. Many reported that depression and anxiety lessened considerably. Others reported that anxiety seemed to disappear entirely.

The outstanding feature about a walking program is that it is so easy. It doesn't require expensive clothing or equipment. Your only special need is a good pair of shoes and the determination to get out there and walk. You can walk alone, with a dog or friend, or with your spouse. In retirement communities walking is usually very popular, not only because of its health aspects but because it provides companionship for those who might otherwise lead lonely lives.

Before you start on the Walk to Health program, you should first check with your physician to make sure that you are fit to do so. After you have obtained your doctor's blessings, you will then need to establish a regular schedule in order to make your health walks a priority.

Ground Rules

Before you begin walking, you will have to follow basic ground rules if you are to get the most out of your walks and at the same time protect your back.

1. Select a suitable pair of walking shoes. Pointed shoes are out, and so are high heels. The shoes should have plenty of cushioning, with a heel elevation of ½ to ¾ of an inch above the sole. The feet should not slide side to side inside the shoes. The shoes should fit snugly, but they should not be tight. If you are in doubt about your choice of shoes, consult a podiatrist.

2. Walk at a brisk pace. What is a brisk pace? If you walk at a pace in which you cannot carry on a conversation without pausing to catch your breath, you are walking too vigorously—slow down. I like to call a brisk pace "conversational walking." Others refer to it as a "talk test."

3. Once you start walking, don't stop until you have finished.

4. Wear comfortable clothing that permits freedom of movement and ventilation.

5. Follow your own schedule, don't advance more than recommended below. If the first walk feels too strenuous, reduce your walking time by 5 minutes a day until you are comfortable.

If you have been habitually inactive for a long period of time, you should be aware of certain signs that indicate to you that you are exceeding your current physical limitations. These may be warning signals, and should any occur while you are on the walking program, stop walking and consult with your physician. Here are the warning signs.

Discomfort in the chest, jaw, neck, or back are signals that you are overextending yourself. Your walk should not produce discomfort. Slow down.

Unusual tiredness, producing a worn-out feeling, after a walk means it was probably done too strenuously. Slow down the pace the next time you venture out.

Light-headedness, dizziness, a noticeably fast heartbeat or a nauseous feeling are other signs that you are overextending yourself.

Difficulty falling asleep at night can also be a warning that you are pushing yourself too hard.

If any of these occur, check with your doctor and describe the symptoms to him.

Here is a progressive series of 10 weekly walk programs that will help guide you step by step along the way. The schedule calls for you to walk every other day. On the days when you are *not* walking, do all 18 of the Y's Healthy Back program exercises.

Before you *do* walk you should always do certain warm-up exercises, and *after* your walk has been completed you will need to do what are called cool-down exercises.

Both warm-up and cool-down exercises will be listed in the first week's schedule and will be referred to as "warm-up" and "cool-down" in subsequent weeks.

The First Week

Do Exercises 1 through 8 from the Y's program.

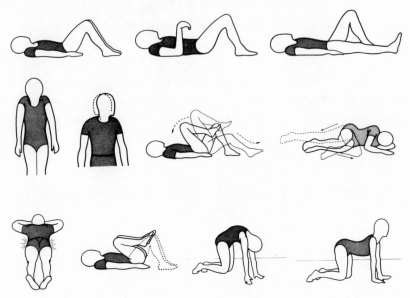

After you have done the eight basic exercises, skip Exercises 9, 10, and 11 and do Exercise 12.

Exercise 12. Sit-up with Feet Secured.

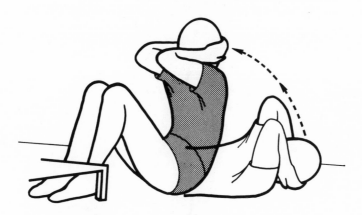

After you do Exercise 12, skip Exercise 13 and do Exercise 14.

Exercise 14. First Hamstring Stretch.

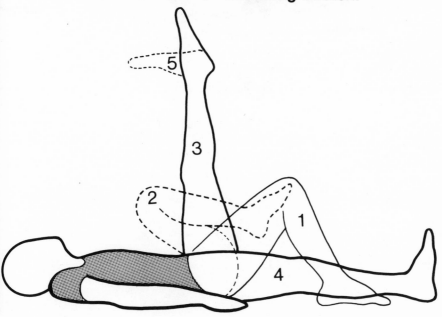

Now do Exercise 15.

Exercise 15. Second Hamstring Stretch.

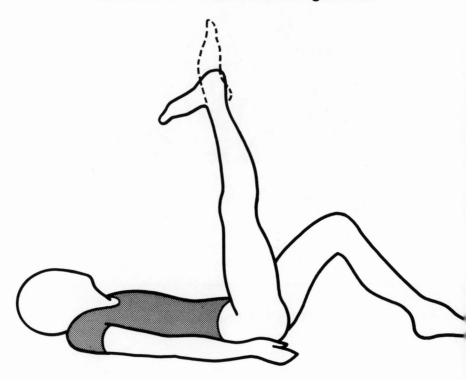

Do Exercise 16.

Exercise 16. Hamstring Stretch, Standing.

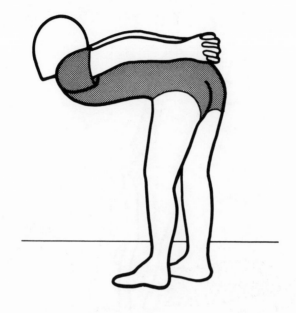

Do Exercise 17.

Exercise 17. Calf Muscle Stretch.

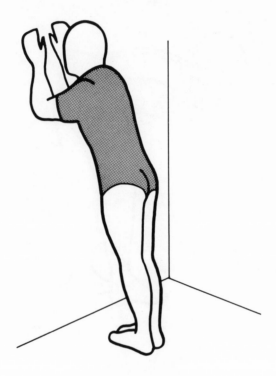

Do Exercise 18.

Exercise 18. Floor Touch (Floor Reach).

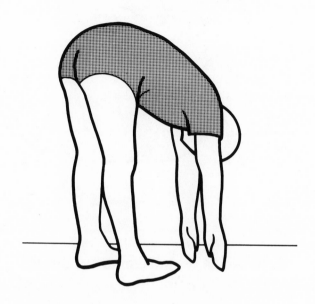

Now walk 15 minutes. Remember, you walk 15 minutes *every other day*, not every day, and on the days when you do not walk, you do the full program of Y's Healthy Back exercises, 1 through 18 and then back down to 1. After you have walked for 15 minutes you perform the cool-down exercises. This consists of doing Exercises 1 through 8 again, just as previously shown.

After doing Exercise 8, the Cat Back, do Exercise 12.

Exercise 12. Sit-up with Feet Secured.

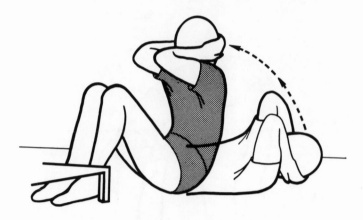

Next, do Exercise 14.

Exercise 14. First Hamstring Stretch.

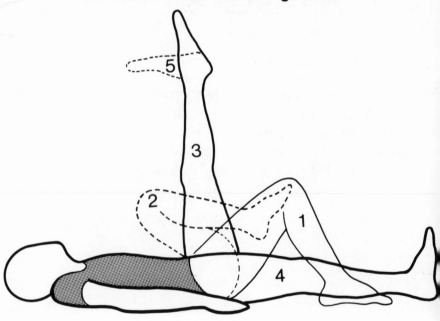

Do Exercise 15.

Exercise 15. Second Hamstring Stretch.

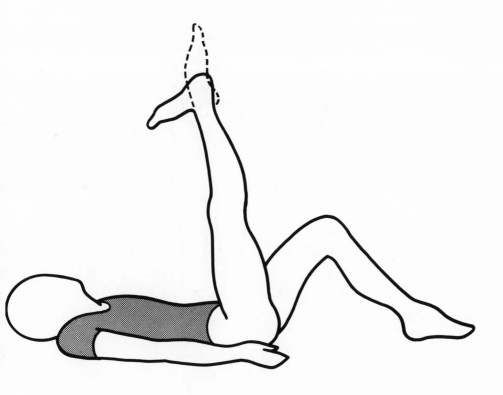

Do Exercise 16.

Exercise 16. Hamstring Stretch, Standing.

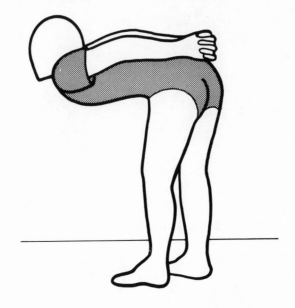

Do Exercise 17.

Exercise 17. Calf Muscle Stretch.

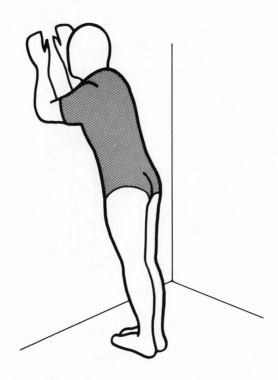

Last, do Exercise 18.

Exercise 18. Floor Touch (Floor Reach).

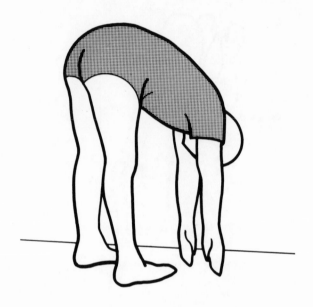

After you have finished the floor touch, do Exercises 6 through 1. That finishes the cool-down. Do the warm-up and cool-down exercises, as shown here, on each day that you do the Walk to Health program. Again, this program takes ten weeks to build up to your potential.

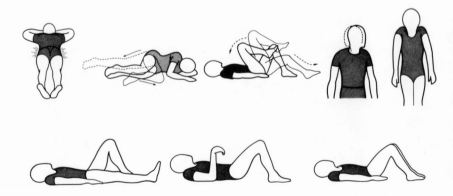

The Second Week

    A. Warm-up Exercises
    B. Walk 20 minutes every other day.
    C. Cool-down Exercises

The Third Week

    A. Warm-up Exercises
    B. Walk 25 minutes every other day.
    C. Cool-down Exercises

The Fourth Week

    A. Warm-up Exercises
    B. Walk 30 minutes every other day.
    C. Cool-down Exercises

The Fifth Week

    A. Warm-up Exercises
    B. Walk 35 minutes every other day.
    C. Cool-down Exercises

The Sixth Week

    A. Warm-up Exercises
    B. Walk 40 minutes every other Day.
    C. Cool-down Exercises

The Seventh Week

  A. Warm-up Exercises
  B. Walk 45 minutes every other day.
  C. Cool-down Exercises

The Eighth Week

  A. Warm-up Exercises
  B. Walk 50 minutes every other day.
  C. Cool-down Exercises

The Ninth Week

  A. Warm-up Exercises
  B. Walk 55 minutes every other day.
  C. Cool-down Exercises

The Tenth Week

  A. Warm-up Exercises
  B. Walk 1 hour every other day.
  C. Cool-down Exercises

Keep on walking. You may want to increase your endurance. As Hippocrates said, "Walking is man's best medicine."

CHAPTER
12
Dynamic Health and Fitness

That which is used develops; that which is not wastes away. This wise statement has been confirmed many times over by modern medical researchers. The human body is a marvelous machine and, unlike other machines, it improves the more you put it to use—within reason, of course. Achieving and maintaining dynamic health and fitness can be a difficult task in an affluent, mechanized society with every so-called "convenience" readily at hand, but you can do it with a progressive exercise program tailored to your needs. If you do not, your body will succumb to the aging process at an accelerated rate.

Some years ago, Dr. Vojin Smodlaka, director of Rehabilitative Medicine at Brooklyn Methodist Hospital, studied various physiological areas of human athletic performance, including stamina. Stamina was measured by cardiovascular endurance, and Dr. Smodlaka, who examined records for the 10,000 meter run and the marathon from the years 1900 to 1960, found that regular distance runners reached their peak of cardiovascular endurance not when they were 18, 26 or 30, but rather when they were 40 years old. Forty is an impressive figure, especially when you compare it with the findings of Dr. Hardin Jones of the University of California at Los Angeles, who measured blood flow through the muscle mass of sedentary American males. He found that the efficiency of the heart to circulate blood in the sedentary male peaks not at 40, not at 30, not even at 26, but at 18. This is shocking. Moreover, he found that if the sedentary male continued his inactive ways, he lost 40 percent of his heart's efficiency to push blood through the muscles by the time he was 26. In cardiovascular terms, he was entering middle age. It is tragic that so many Americans settle for such a low level of cardiovascular fitness when their potential for dynamic health and fitness is so enormous.

What is the result when people fail to exercise, and to build up stamina? They gradually fall prey to stress and lapse into a state of negative health balance. They succumb to avoidable sickness and to premature aging, manifested by overweight, high blood pressure, high neuro-muscular tension, high pulse rate, low adreno–cortical reserve, low breathing capacity, low muscle strength and flexibility, low heart strength, and low emotional stability. They become ready victims of low back pain, ulcers, colitis, tension headaches, nervous disorders, obesity, impotence and cardiovascular disease. The only way to fend off the sinister but subtle influence of the sedentary life is to become and remain active by doing purposeful physical exercise on a regular basis.

In addition to the Y's Healthy Back program, you should also do exercises to improve your stamina. The best exercises involve the rhythmical and continuous use of the leg muscles, as in walking, jogging, running, cycling and swimming. The large muscles of the body, particularly the leg muscles, act as auxiliary pumps to the heart. They help keep the blood moving and they are crucial to the health of the cardiovascular wall. To a lesser, but still significant extent, rhythmical and continuous use of the arms performs the same function. Look at the long lives orchestra conductors, such as Arturo Toscanini, Arthur Fiedler, and Sir Thomas Beecham have led. In fact, people who have lost their legs are instructed to exercise their arms so they can build up stamina. The arms and legs are not just extremities of our bodies to facilitate eating or getting up and down the stairs; they are a vital part of the human body, in which everything works better when everything works together.

I say this because some of you were inactive before you took the Y's Way to a Healthy Back program. You are better for being active. In addition to doing the Y's exercises, you should take up the walking program described in Chapter 11. If you were active previously in sports, follow the program given in Chapter 10.

No matter which course you follow, bear this in mind: *the older you get, the more you should exercise, but less intensely.* Let's examine this by age categories. If you are between 20 and 30 years of age, you can maintain a fairly good level of fitness if you devote two days a week to intense physical workouts lasting an hour each.

If you are between 30 and 40, you should workout three days a week for an hour each time, but not as intensely as a 20- to 30-year old.

If you are 40 to 50 years of age, you should exercise for an hour every other day, but less intensely than you did in the previous decade.

If you are between 50 and 60, you should exercise for an hour at least six days a week, but less intensely than the 40 to 50 year olds.

If you are past 60, you should exercise every day, but less intensely than the 50 to 60 year olds.

In short, to forestall the aging process, increase the frequency of exercise but decrease the intensity as you grow older. By doing so you'll find that you look younger and feel better than your peers who don't.

CHAPTER

13

Dealing with Stress;

*Some Myths,
Avoiding Bad Back Habits,
and Relieving Sudden
Back Stress*

I would now like to discuss stress because not everyone understands what stress is, and how it can affect your muscles and your back. In 1936, Dr. Hans Selye, a pioneer in the field, defined stress as "the nonspecific response of the body to any demand." A demand or "stressor" can be any one of a number of things, external or internal, such as a noise, a fight with a spouse, glare from a light, a deadline to be met, concern over illness of a family member or friend, difficult working conditions, a neighbor's barking dog, fear of losing your job, and so on. Everyone alive experiences stress. What you must learn to do is deal with stress. In his book, *Managing Stress,* Dr. Leon J. Warshaw, a member of the Y's Medical Advisory Board, devotes part of a chapter to backache, which along with alcoholism, drug abuse, mass psychogenic illness and absenteeism, is a reaction to stress. "Backache (low back pain) is an extremely common stress reaction that is particularly burdensome to both the employee and the work organization," Dr. Warshaw writes. "Its exact incidence is not known, but it has been said that 80 percent of the population will experience at least one disabling episode during adult life. Most backaches are attributed to an acute strain or trauma resulting from an attempt to lift something or an injudicious movement. Careful investigation, however, frequently reveals that the precipitating incident was coincidental, the real cause being chronic tension, stiffness, and weakness of key postural muscles induced by stress. Especially in sedentary individuals in whom these muscles are weakened by inactivity, the tension itself can produce a soreness but, more important, it also leaves the muscles vulnerable to injury by a sudden or strenuous movement."

If the initial cause is not corrected, episodes are recurrent, and the person suffering from low back pain gets on what is called the treatment treadmill. "X-rays are taken and, in 20 to 60 percent of cases, depending on how rigorously they are interpreted, they show structural defects or evidence of 'arthritis' that have been associated with 'instability' and pain in the spine (actually they are found with similar frequency in individuals without pain)," Dr. Warshaw writes. "The patient is hospitalized for several weeks of traction therapy, usually with a diagnosis of 'disc disease.' Consultations are arranged with orthopedists, neurologists, neurosurgeons, etc. Special X-rays and other diagnostic procedures are performed and nerve blocks and other kinds of injections may be tried. When these fail, surgery to correct the structural defect is usually advised."

And what happens when the patient emerges from surgery and still suffers from low back pain? There is additional stress and the situation deteriorates rapidly. A brochure published by the Memorial Hospital Medical Center of Long Beach, California, reports that "the problem can become chronic and, at its worst, catastrophic. Absences from work multiply or become prolonged. Repeated hospitalization and surgery may become more and more frequent. Marital and home life may deteriorate. Psychological and emotional conflicts may become as severe as the physical problem."

Some sufferers from stress may require psychological counseling. Whether or not you do, the Y's exercises can help you to deal with stress. As Dr. Warshaw writes, "Almost every form of exercise will act as an antidote to stress reactions if practiced regularly. Perhaps the only exceptions are competitive sports and games for those people who become obsessive about achieving a standard of performance or compulsive about winning."

Dr. Warshaw notes that the primary approach to the problem of low back pain "requires recognition of the fundamental role in its genesis played by stress and muscle deficiency and the opportunity to control those factors in the work setting that are inordinately stressful. But since stressors in their personal and home lives are equally, if not more, troublesome for most individuals, an approach is needed that will relieve their discomfort and increase their capacity to tolerate stress without initiating the back-pain syndrome. Such an approach is the Y's Way to a Healthy Back program."

I did not quote the last sentence to give the Y a pat on the back, so to speak, but to emphasize that the Y's program can help you to deal with stress, and if your back pain is related to stress, you can avoid the pain by doing the Healthy Back exercises. A perfect case in point: Dr. Kraus and I both know a free-lance magazine writer who is always under the gun traveling and meeting deadlines. I'll call him Ned. He is really one wound-up character. Some years ago, Ned was asked to do a major article on back pain, and in the course of doing his reporting on the subject, he heard about the Kraus–Weber Tests. Intrigued by what he heard, he arranged to interview Dr. Kraus. When the interview was just about finished, Ned asked Dr. Kraus if he could take the Kraus–Weber Tests. The doctor readily agreed. Ned passed all of them with flying colors except the sixth, the floor touch.

"Your hamstrings and calf muscles are very tense," said the doctor. "You ought to start exercising."

"I can't because of my work," said Ned. "I'm on the go all the time. Rat-tat-tat-tat. If I don't put myself under pressure, I feel guilty. I have to write to take care of my family. I make only what I receive from writing. I get no salary. So I have to keep hustling all the time. If I'm not under stress, I don't feel normal."

"You should deal with the stress," Dr. Kraus said. "You lack flexibility, and you should start exercising. If I have ever seen a candidate for low back pain, you're it."

"Thanks for the advice, doctor," Ned said, "but I'm too busy to do any exercises. Your Kraus–Weber Tests are interesting, and if I ever do suffer a back problem, I'll come to you."

Two years later, Ned called Dr. Kraus for an appointment. Several days later, Ned came in for an examination. "You were right, doctor," he said. "My back feels as though someone hit it with an axe." He said that he had been having a difficult time writing an article at home, and to get over his mental block at the typewriter he had decided to take a break and mow the lawn. Ned had an old-fashioned pusher mower. "Some twigs got stuck in the blades," he said, "and you know me, doctor. Instead of stopping to pick the twigs out of the blades, I decided to give the mower a push so the blades would chop them up. I gave a push, but the mower wouldn't move. I gave another push, this one much harder, and suddenly a horrible pain ripped across my back. I fell to my knees in agony, and my wife, who had been watching from inside the house, ran out to see what was wrong with me. She thought I was having a heart attack. I told her about the pain in my back, and she helped me hobble into the house and get into bed. The next day when the pain hadn't gone away, I called you."

Dr. Kraus treated Ned and put him on an exercise program. It took three months for the pain to disappear completely, and during that time Ned missed out on a couple of well-paying assignments because he could not travel. Since then, he has kept up with his daily exercises and, as he told me recently, "I don't do them just to keep back pain away. I do them because I have to do them. If I miss just one day, I can feel tightness in my calf muscles and hamstrings and I feel under stress mentally. The exercises get rid of the stress and give me a good feeling, a lift, a sense of mental well-being."

Bad Back Habits

Besides dealing with stress, you may need to correct some personal habits or alter the way you live. Following are a number of "little things" that can induce back or neck pain.

Using the telephone. Never cradle it between your neck and shoulder. This can bring on neck and shoulder pain.

Reading. Don't hold your muscles in a forced position by holding a newspaper too close or too far away so you can read it. This can bring on back and neck strain. Maybe you need new eyeglasses.

Work positions. Avoid maintaining a certain position for too long. Get up, walk around, change positions.

Chairs. There is no miracle chair that is good for everyone. The proper selection will depend on your particular build. Firm surfaces are best. This also includes adequate thigh support and a seat high enough so that knees and hips form right angles with feet on the floor.

Driving. When driving long distances, stop the car every hour or so and take a short walk. This will greatly relieve the strain of sitting in one position too long.

Shoes. Select shoes that are wide and comfortable, with slight cushioning. Avoid exaggerated heels which shorten calf and hamstring muscles. High heels will throw your weight toward the forward part of the foot causing back strain.

Shoulder bags. Shoulder bags, photographic gear carriers and attache' cases can be risky. Heavy loads should be balanced on both shoulders. If weight cannot be evenly divided, shift the weight from side to side regularly to relieve undue strain on one side.

Lifting objects. Lift with your legs, not with your back. This is a good rule to follow. Bend the knees, lift the object and tighten the stomach as you lift by pulling in and up. For light objects, such as bending to pick up a piece of paper, there is no harm in doing what is called a "dead lift," with the knees straight. Many people have trouble in attempting to lift large objects from car trunks. Very often you may be tense from a long drive and stiff from sitting too long; to avoid trouble, drag the heavy object to the rim of the trunk and gradually ease it out.

Girdles and corsets. A girdle or a corset can restrain the natural movements of the trunk and impede bending. As Dr. Kraus says, "If a woman is in good condition, she does not need to wear a girdle. If she is not in good condition, she should try to build up her stomach muscles so she can get along without support."

Brassieres. Narrow shoulder straps can force the wearer into a rigid position and make muscles tense and painful in the shoulders and upper back.

Nightclothes. Nightgowns and pajamas should be loose fitting so that they do not restrict movement when sleeping.

Mattresses. Choose a firm sleeping surface, such as a hard mattress set directly on a wooden frame to prevent muscle stiffness. All muscles have what is called a "jelling time"—the time it takes them to stiffen from the strain of staying in one position too long. The older you are, the shorter your jelling time. The object is to keep shifting position. Soft surfaces tend to mold themselves to the body's contours so you move much less during your sleep. A hard surface will require you to change positions more often, thus minimizing stiffness.

Pillows. Avoid the use of foam rubber. It is one of the primary culprits causing neck stiffness. Choose, instead, a pillow filled with feather down or manufactured fiber.

Sleeping positions. Sleep any way that is comfortable. If your accustomed position is on the stomach and you are having discomfort, a pillow placed under your hips can help. If sleeping on your back is causing pain, try slipping a pillow under your knees for relief.

Relieving a Sudden Back Attack

If you happen to suffer a sudden attack of low back pain or muscle spasm, here are some simple methods that can help you obtain relief. First, have a family member or friend soak a towel in very hot water. Next, lie on your stomach. Your helper should then wring out the towel and place it immediately over the painful area. The heat will dissipate quickly, so repeated applications will be required. It's the heat shock that helps. Keep this up for 15 minutes. Then, if you are already doing the exercises in the Y's Healthy Back program, do the relaxation exercises, 1 through 6, and back again to 1, as described in Chapter 4. While you are doing the exercises, your helper can put on a glove and massage the painful area with ice cubes. Ethyl chloride spray is even more effective than ice massage, but it is obtainable only by perscription and it must be used carefully because it can cause frost bite.

George Pasiuk, a former Y Healthy Back instructor, was all alone when he suffered a muscle spasm in his lower back while he was moving furniture. George, who was in otherwise excellent shape, immediately took a very hot shower and did the relaxation exercises, 1 through 6 and back down to 1. He did this for the next two days, and by the end of the second day he was fine.

If you are subjected to repeated episodes of sudden back pain, you may have "triggerpoints" which require treatment by a physician. Triggerpoints are nodules of degenerated muscle tissue that can literally trigger pain and spasm. They can occur in different parts of the body—so-called tennis elbow is usually caused by triggerpoints—and they are commonly found in the lower back muscles. Triggerpoints can only be eliminated by the use of needles—injections. Dr. Kraus describes the technique in his book, *Sports Injuries*. Unfortunately, most physicians are not aware of triggerpoints and how they should be treated, so if need be ask your doctor to refer you to a physician who is knowledgeable about triggerpoint therapy.

CHAPTER

14

Medical Research on Low Back Pain and the Y's Program

What we know now about the causes of low back pain is the result of research by a number of physicians and investigators particularly in the field of physical medicine and rehabilitation. Dr. Hans Kraus of New York City has done outstanding research in this field. As the late Dr. Frederick Seitz, President of the prestigious National Academy of Sciences, once remarked, "Every individual who has suffered backache should become familiar with the principles and corrective measures to which Dr. Kraus has devoted so much of his career."

A pioneer advocate of physical fitness, in 1954 Dr. Kraus was instrumental in persuading President Eisenhower to launch what is now known as the President's Council on Physical Fitness and Sports and in 1980 he was the recipient of the council's Distinguished Service Award. Dr. Kraus is the author of numerous medical papers, three books for the medical profession, *Principles and Practices of Therapeutic Exercise, Hypokinetic Disease* (with Dr. Wilhelm Raab) and *Clinical Treatment of Back and Neck Pain,* and two excellent popular works, *Backache: Stress and Tension* and *Sports Injuries.*

Now in his 70s, Dr. Kraus has led a remarkable life both as a person and as a physician. He grew up in Trieste and Zurich where James Joyce served as the family English tutor. A life-long sportsman, Dr. Kraus at one time boxed and raced motorcycles.

145

He is an expert rock and mountain climber and downhill and cross country skier. In 1974, he was elected to the Ski Hall of Fame for his services to the United States Olympic ski team and for his years as an official advisory physician of the National Ski Patrol. As a doctor, he found his true calling in the early 1930s while serving as a resident in surgery at the University of Vienna hospital. It was then that he began to realize the value of exercise and its effect upon the muscular system, particularly in re-habilitating patients who were recovering from fractures. As a resident, he had to review the case histories of hundreds of patients who had suffered wrist fractures, and in so doing he discovered that those who recovered best were those who exer-cised the most after suffering a fracture. Their rate of rehabilita-tion was far better and more rapid than those patients who had done little or no exercise, regardless of the severity of the frac-ture. Given this finding, the university hospital began checking on rehabilitation of patients who had suffered other fractures, and the same pattern emerged. Those who had exercised recovered more quickly than those who had not. As a result, the hospital instituted special exercise programs to rehabilitate the muscular flexibility and strength of all patients who had been bedridden for any length of time. The program was very successful.

Soon afterward, Dr. Kraus happened to be talking with a close friend, a coach named Heinz Kowalski, who was President of the Austrian Sports Teachers Association. In the course of the conversation it occurred to Dr. Kraus that although Kowalski sent many patients with fractures to the hospital, he had never sent anyone to the hospital with a muscle strain or ligament injury. He asked Kowalski why. Kowalski said the doctors at the hospital would only put them in a plaster of Paris cast, or splints, and thus immobilize them. When Dr. Kraus responded that the only way to heal such injuries was to impose long rest from movement, Kowalski reminded the doctor that he, Kowalski, came from a circus family, and whenever anyone in the circus suffered a sprain or strain, they had to keep working or they'd be out of a job. Kowalski said that an injured performer would soak a towel in alcohol, wrap it around the injury and then expose the towel to a steady cloud of hot steam. This numbed the injury, and the performer could begin to move the limb. After doing this several times a day, the performer was usually able to get back to work after only a day or two.

Dr. Kraus began to experiment with the Kowalski method. It was successful but cumbersome, and he began to experiment with chemicals that could produce numbness. Finally, he decided to use ethyl chloride spray, which physicians were then employing as a local anesthetic when making small incisions. The ethyl chloride, when combined with gentle movement of the injured area, contributed to the rapid recovery of patients whom Dr. Kraus treated for either sprains or strains. In 1932, he presented a paper on the use of ethyl chloride spray at the Vienna Academy of Physicians, and a correspondent for the American Medical Association who was present was so fascinated by it that an abstract of the paper was published in the *Journal of the American Medical Association.*

On a visit to the United States in 1934, Dr. Kraus demonstrated his techniques at New York Columbia Presbyterian Hospital, and when he settled in New York in 1938, Drs. William Darrach and Clay Ray Murray, orthopedic surgeons at Columbia University's College of Physicians and Surgeons, asked him to continue his research and clinical practice in physical medicine and rehabilitation while he was serving as Assistant Surgeon because it was so valuable. In 1940, Dr. Kraus and Dr. Sonja Weber began working in the posture clinic of Columbia Presbyterian Hospital, studying children who had posture problems, and their work was to have extraordinary significance for back pain sufferers everywhere. In 1944, Dr. Kraus was appointed to the hospital's Department of Physical Medicine and Rehabilitation. In 1947, he was appointed Associate Professor of Physical Medicine and Rehabilitation at the New York University Medical School.

The great majority of the children in the clinic were considered normal except for poor posture, and Drs. Kraus and Weber

spent a great deal of time examining the youngsters, photograph-
ing them and conducting other studies in an effort to assess their
condition. From their observations, Drs. Kraus and Weber came
up with the hypothesis that muscular inability to move properly
was the root cause of poor posture, and to test their hypothesis
they decided to measure the flexibility and strength of the key
muscle groups used to hold the body erect. Several years of work
went into their efforts, and when it was done, they had devised
a battery of six tests—the Kraus–Weber Tests—shown in Chapter 2. The tests were designed to reveal which key muscle groups
were weak or tense. By having youngsters take the tests, Drs.
Kraus and Weber could readily understand why children allowed
their shoulders to slump, let their stomachs stick out, or exhibited
other examples of poor posture. The two doctors then gave each
child prescribed exercises to do. Those who did them regularly
usually improved, while those who started the exercises and
stopped them soon displayed poor posture again.

Drs. Kraus and Weber spent four years working with the
children in the posture clinic, and just as their research was
nearing completion in 1944, Dr. Barbara Stimson asked them to
take part in a group clinic she had organized at Columbia
Presbyterian, under the auspices of Drs. Clay Ray Murray and
William Darrach, to investigate the causes of low back pain. Drs.
Kraus and Weber joined a number of specialists, including inter-
nists, neurologists, neurosurgeons and orthopedic surgeons, in
examining and evaluating some 3,000 adult patients suffering
from low back pain. All the patients underwent a thorough medical examination which included X-rays and laboratory tests. In
addition, Drs. Kraus and Weber gave them the Kraus–Weber
Tests to determine the flexibility and strength of their key posture muscles. An orthopedic surgeon, Dr. Sawnie Gaston, then
reviewed the data and concluded that 83 percent of the 3,000
patients, almost 2500 of them, did not show any specific lesion,
disease, or anomaly such as a ruptured disc. Instead, this 83
percent suffered from low back pain because their muscles were
weak and/or tense.

At this point, Drs. Kraus and Weber prescribed exercises for these patients, the results were very dramatic. A total of 65 percent of the patients who did the prescribed exercises reported they had no pain whatever, 26 percent reported only occasional discomfort, and nine percent had no relief. Drs. Kraus and Weber then followed 233 of the patients for approximately eight years and, as Dr. Kraus wrote in *Clinical Treatment of Back and Neck Pain,* "It was found that the symptoms of these patients diminished with increased muscle strength and flexibility and reoccurred when they stopped their therapeutic exercise or physical activities and returned to their former state of weakness and inflexibility. Generally speaking, a very strong association existed and continued between muscle deficiency on the one hand and pain and disability on the other."

Drs. Kraus and Weber made another interesting finding: tight and stiff back muscles responded to limbering and stretching exercises, but the response varied, depending on the tension status of the individual. Since then, research has shown that people can become tense for different reasons. For one it may be money worries, for another the impending visit of a mother-in-law, and for yet another the blare of a neighbor's record player. This is the raging, tearing 20th century, when future shock is now. Most people now lead tremendously overstimulated lives, starting from the time they get up in the morning and head off to work. The commuter on the train worries about whether he will get to the city on time for an appointment. The commuter who drives to work becomes irritated by a traffic tie-up, or the rude driver who cuts him off at the light. The housewife finds that the washing machine won't work. At the office, an angry boss can make you tense, and the boss gets tense when the typist who is always taking a coffee break doesn't get that important letter out. All this is part and parcel of hectic 20th century living and unless you take the time to exercise to relieve the constant assaults, tension will build up in your muscles and make them very tight. In the 1920s, Dr. Walter B. Cannon of Harvard, a noted physiologist and the author of *The Wisdom of the Body,* studied the reactions of a number of animals to irritation. The animals reacted with a rise in blood pressure, an outpouring of adrenaline, increased respiration, a rise in blood sugar and the tensing of muscles. In the wild, the animals would have responded by attacking or fleeing, the so-called "fight or flight" response. The same happens to humans, but in this day and age you can't react by punching someone or running away and, as Dr. Kraus notes in *Clinical Treatment of Back and Neck Pain,* "In our lives, where neither is possible, this complex of reactions is stopped at its peak and cannot complete its physiological course. It backfires and becomes pathogenic."

Repeated tension shortens muscles. A German physiologist named Tiegel showed that repeated tensing of a muscle results in loss of length in contracture—and shortened muscles lack elasticity or give. "Once the muscle tightness has reached a sufficiently high level, and lack of physical activity has weakened the tense muscles," Dr. Kraus writes, "the stage is set for the first episode of back pain. Even so small an act as picking up a paper or pencil may precipitate the first attack, which leaves the muscles weakened and more stiffened—ready for the next episode of pain which in turn will compound the symptoms."

Drs. Kraus and Weber continued their research on back pain. In the years following World War II, back pain was becoming a commonplace affliction in affluent America, and the two doctors began to wonder if the very life style of Americans might be at the root of the problem. In 1947, they tested their hypothesis by comparing healthy American children, who were growing up in a society dominated by mechanization, with healthy youngsters in less affluent surroundings in Austria, Switzerland and Italy. The American and European youngsters were between the ages of six and 16, and in total 5,000 were tested in the U.S., while 3,000 were tested in Europe. All were tested the same way: they were asked to do the six exercises in the Kraus–Weber Tests.

The results were startling. Almost 58 percent of the American youngsters failed one or more of the six Kraus–Weber Tests, while less than nine percent of the European children failed. (Follow-up research revealed that in the next decade the rate of failure almost doubled in Austria as that country prospered and mechanized.)

Dr. Kraus wrote about the muscular deficiency of American youngsters, and in 1954 the Amateur Athletic Union reprinted an article that he had written for the *New York State Journal of Medicine*. John B. Kelly, Sr., a wealthy Philadelphian and a former national sculling champion (and the father of the late Princess Grace of Monaco) happened to read it. Kelly found the findings so disturbing that he passed the article on to Senator James Duff of Pennsylvania, and Senator Duff brought it to the attention of President Dwight Eisenhower.

As a result, President Eisenhower invited Dr. Kraus to a luncheon meeting at the White House. The guest list included such sports stars as Willie Mays and Tony Trabert, but as *Sports Illustrated* reported in a major article entitled, "The Report that Shocked the President," this was "one day the stars sat back" as Dr. Kraus reported on the findings. The President called the problem a serious one; it was, in fact, even more alarming than he had imagined, and he started the President's Council on Youth Fitness and Sports.

The Kraus–Weber Tests proved to be of value to adults of all ages in analyzing the causes of low back pain—and in predicting who was likely to suffer from it. Over the years, Dr. Kraus has continued to do research, practice, write, and speak out about the problem, and we at the National YMCA believe ourselves fortunate that the Y has been able to avail itself of Hans Kraus' insights into the problem—and its solution.

The Y's Way to a Healthy Back program owes its inception to Stanley Newhouse, Chairman of the Physical Fitness Council of the YMCA of Greater New York. As head of a financial planning firm, he was well aware of the actuarial figures showing the number of medical claims based on back problems. At the time, in 1973, I was the executive for Health and Physical Education for the Metropolitan YMCA of Greater New York, and Newhouse asked me to investigate the possibility of developing an exercise program for the prevention and treatment of low back pain based on the principles and methods of Dr. Kraus.

I was well aware of Dr. Kraus' work in the field, and I went to see him. In our initial meeting, he was interested but cautious, and he said he would think about what he might do. Several months later, Dr. Kraus and I met again. He said that he had thought about what the Y might do, and was now enthusiastic about starting a program for the Y. Enthusiastic is a mild word. On his own, Dr. Kraus had lined up a panel of distinguished physicians (five of whom had treated Presidents of the United States) to serve as members of a medical advisory board. Dr. Kraus noted that the need for a nationwide back program was obvious. He had been speaking and writing about the problem for almost 20 years, but even if every lay person heeded his word, physicians in general were not responding and there was no way he could treat everyone who sought to see him for private treatment. The only way low back pain could be treated and prevented (on a mass basis, he said) was through a mass exercise program throughout the United States. Nothing had been done in this line in this country, but he pointed out that a number of European nations, including West Germany and the Soviet Union, had established reconditioning centers. In the Soviet Union, at least according to the Russian claim, some five million patients a year were undergoing reconditioning treatment for hypokinetic diseases. "We like to think that we're way ahead of the Soviet Union," Dr. Kraus said, "but when you consider the fact that the Soviet Union has nowhere near the prosperous and underexercised populace we have in the United States, you have to wonder why we have taken no action!"

In West Germany, Dr. Kraus continued, great progress had been made by the establishment of reconditioning centers, and inasmuch as socio-economic conditions in West Germany were very similar to those in the United States, the West German centers could serve as models for this country. For instance, Dr. Peter Beckmann had set up a reconditioning center in Ohlstadt, Bavaria which was so successful in treating physically inactive people that 15 more reconditioning centers were soon begun. "The YMCA might be the very agency to use in the United States for mass treatment and prevention of low back pain," Dr. Kraus said, "and we ought to test this by starting a pilot program to see if it can be done through the Y."

I agreed, and we set about planning a feasibility or pilot study to take place in the spring of 1974. Stan Newhouse was pleased at the news, and I selected a dozen YMCA physical directors to join me in being trained by Dr. Kraus. Our pilot program began in May. We were interested in determining two things: (1) whether or not the public would respond and (2) to see if it was feasible to direct a program on such a large scale. In our first pilot program we enrolled 63 people with low back pain. By September a total of 216 people had taken and completed the program. We were elated by the response and success. Our efforts proved that properly trained instructors could help people overcome low back pain problems and show them how to avoid future episodes. Our efforts also showed that people with low back pain would avail themselves of a program specifically tailored for them. Word of the success of the initial programs spread quickly throughout the northeast, and a number of Y's in the region sought to join the program. In October of 1974, we selected and trained another 24 physical educators, all from Y's in small towns and medium-sized cities. We wanted to see whether the program would go over there as it had in New York, with its large population base. It did, and after we reported the success in the *Journal of Physical Education* in February of 1975, we were inundated with requests for the program from Y's all across the country. Shortly thereafter, the National Board of the YMCAs unanimously endorsed the Y's Way to a Healthy Back program as an official National YMCA program offering.

Dr. Kraus and I then personally trained 300 physical educators across the country. We visited key cities representing geographical regions of the Y and brought future instructors to two-day theoretic and practical seminars so that they became thoroughly familiar with the exercise program and its medical philosophy.

By now the program was in such demand that it was impossible for Dr. Kraus and I to train each new instructor personally, so we chose 26 highly qualified Y professional educators to become instructor–trainers for other physical educators who would conduct the program. As new instructors joined the program nationwide, Dr. Kraus and I wrote instruction manuals and program guidelines to make certain that, as the program expanded, we could maintain the highest levels of quality control and standards of safety. We made it an absolute rule that any person enrolling in the program had to obtain a physician's approval beforehand. I cannot emphasize this point enough.

By mid-1976 our 26 instructor–trainers had trained several hundred YMCA personnel in the conduct of the Y's Way to a Healthy Back program, and we requested that all participating instructors throughout this country and Canada send to my office participant data on at least one class annually. We did this to ascertain instructor effectiveness and to build a statistical base for study and analysis to make certain we were as effective as we could be.

Dr. Kraus, Dr. Sawnie Gaston, former associate professor of Clinical Orthopedic Surgery at Columbia University's College of Physicians and Surgeons, and I analyzed the first set of preliminary data that was returned from Y's across the country, and in July of 1977 we published our first article in the *New York State Journal of Medicine*. There we reported on the results of a back pain questionnaire filled out by 421 subjects who had completed the Y's Way to a Healthy Back program. We scored the preliminary results as follows:

Excellent response: all pain disappeared, can do almost everything, 29.27 percent.

Good response: much less pain, can do most things, 36.23 percent.

Fair response: less pain, can do more things, 25.23 percent.

Poor response: slightly less pain or no improvement, 9.27 percent.

Ninety percent of the participants had at least improved. We believed these preliminary statistics fully justified the purpose of the program, and we concluded the article by writing, "The success of this program is assured by (1) the integrity of its concept, (2) its implementation by the YMCA, and (3) the endorsement of the medical profession."

We had a two-fold purpose in writing the article. First, we wanted to let physicians know of the success and availability of the program, and second, local Y's could use reprints of the article to establish a connection with doctors in the community. At present, local Y's have distributed more than 100,000 reprints of the article.

In 1981 we conducted a special study of 710 subjects who had undergone a total of 921 back operations. These were people who, following surgery, still had pain. We found that depending on the frequency and duration of the Y's exercises, 65–91 percent reported a reduction in the frequency and severity of their back pain.

In March of 1982, we concluded the computer survey program of 11,809 subjects which showed that 80.7 percent of them experienced improvement after taking the Y's Healthy Back program.

At present, 1,000 Y's in the United States, 58 in Canada, and 12 in Australia offer the six-week program throughout the course of the year. The modest fee, which is set by the local Y giving the program, generally costs a Y member only $50 and a non-member $70. In 1982, about 40,000 people took part in the program as individuals. That figure does not include thousands of others who will take the program on the premises of their employer. In recent years, the YMCA has contracted with a growing number of companies and government agencies—ranging from the Detroit Police Department (54 percent of the disability cases in the 6,000 member force was attributed to back problems) to Polaroid—to conduct the six-week program on their premises. For example, in April 1981, the Y began offering the program to any of IBM's 190,000 employees (plus members of their immediate families and company retirees) at 294 company facilities across the country. IBM contracted with the Y after we ran test programs at three IBM plants in different parts of the country.

IBM and numerous other companies are interested and are

becoming involved with the Y's program because back pain and disability are widespread problems. These are noted in Appendix I. Several years ago Massachusetts Mutual Life Insurance Co. reported that a bad back was the number one cause of claims in disability income policies, followed by fractures, digestive disorders, and heart and circulatory ailments. There are no definitive dollars and cents figures on what low back pain costs the economy nationally—estimates run as high as several billions of dollars—but the New York Telephone Company, which has made it standard practice to identify and computerize the reasons for employee absenteeism, calculates that out-of-whack backs cost the company $4 million a year. Recently, New York Telephone signed a contract with the Y after the company medical department was impressed by two trial back programs we ran. Under the contract, we trained two members of the company to serve as instructors, and New York Telephone agreed to share all data with us when the company evaluates the effects of the program on absenteeism.

The Abitibi Price Paper Company mill in St. Catharine's, Ontario, Canada, contracted with the local Y for the Healthy Back program to be run on plant premises. When it was over, the company tracked 19 employees. The year before those 19 employees enrolled in the program, they had paid 40 visits to the dispensary because of back pain. The year following the program, they made only 21 visits to the dispensary.

The Canadian Life Assurance Company contracted with the Toronto Y for the Healthy Back program, and later on in a special issue of the *Ontario Workmen's Compensation Report*, the company calculated that it had saved $200,000 annually as a result and urged other companies to get in touch with the Y.

Many insurance companies are very interested in the Y's Way to a Healthy Back program. In fact, more than 50 insurance companies will now share the cost with a policy holder who participates in the Y program. These companies include such giants as Aetna Life and Casualty, Bankers Life, Connecticut General, Firemen's Fund, Hartford Insurance, Kemper, Liberty

Mutual, and Prudential. Moreover, nine Blue Cross/Blue Shield plans have done the same (a full list of participating insurance companies and Blue Cross/Blue Shield plans is given in Appendices II and III), as have state compensation boards in California, Nevada, Massachusetts, Oregon, and Ohio.

Recently, YMCA's in Chile, Israel, and Mexico have contacted us to start the programs in their countries.

APPENDIX I

Businesses, Hospitals, and Unions that have Contracted with YMCAs for Employee Programs

1. Abitibi Paper Co., Ltd., St. Catharine's, Ontario, Canada
2. Addison's Cadillac, Toronto, Ontario, Canada
3. Air Products & Chemicals, Inc., Allentown, Pennsylvania
4. Alexian Brothers Hospital, San Jose, California
5. Atlas Crankshaft Co., Mansfield, Ohio
6. Armco Steel Corp., Cincinnati, Ohio and Middletown, Ohio
7. Avco Systems, Wilmington, Massachusetts
8. Avco Lycoming, Stratford, Connecticut
9. AT&T Long Lines Division, Bernardsville, New Jersey; Pittsfield, Massachusetts; Newark, New Jersey; Princeton, New Jersey; White Plains, New York; Stratford, Connecticut; Boston, Massachusetts
10. Bailey Control Co., Wickcliff, Ohio
11. Ball Company, Denver, Colorado
12. Bell Telephone Co., Council Bluff, Iowa; Omaha, Nebraska; Cincinnati, Ohio
13. British Columbia Hospital Employees, British Columbia, Canada
14. British Columbia Hydro-Electric, Vancouver, British Columbia, Canada

15. British Columbia Telephone Co., British Columbia, Canada
16. Canadian Gypsum Co., Toronto, Ontario, Canada
17. Canadian Life Assurance Co., Toronto, Ontario, Canada
18. Charles Machine Works, Perry, Oklahoma
19. Coca Cola Co., Salinas, California
20. Commonwealth Edison Co., Joliet, Illinois
21 Consumers Power Co., Grand Rapids, Michigan
22. Dana Corp., Reading, Pennsylvania
23. Draper Laboratories, Cambridge, Massachusetts
24. Erie Hospital, Erie, Pennsylvania
25. FMC Corp., Pocatello, Idaho
26. Farmington Insurance Group Office, Michigan
27. Firestone Tire, Des Moines, Iowa
28. Ford Aeronautics, Newport Beach, California
29. Forest Oil Co., Corpus Christi, Texas
30. General Electric Co., Stratford, Connecticut
31. Grand Valley Manufacturing Co., Titusville, Pennsylvania
32. Green Manufacturing Co., Racine, Wisconsin
33. Harding Jones Paper Co., Cincinnati, Ohio
34. Harsco Corp., Harrisburg, Pennsylvania; Rochester, Massachusetts; Portland, Oregon; Nashville, Tennessee; Plant City, Florida
35. Hayes Dara Ltd., Thorold, Ontario, Canada
36. Heilmans Brewery, St. Joseph, Missouri
37. Hoffman La Roche, Nutley, New Jersey
38. Honeywell Corporation, Phoenix, Arizona and Rockford, Illinois
39. Houston Forest Products, Houston, British Columbia, Canada
40. Houston Health Center, Houston, British Columbia, Canada
41. Hughes Corporation, Van Nuys, California
42. IBM, available in 294 IBM facilities
43. In-Sink-Erator, Racine, Wisconsin
44. Irwin Toys, Toronto, Ontario, Canada
45. J.I. Case Co., Racine, Wisconsin
46. John Deere, Des Moines, Iowa

47. Johnson's Wax Co., Racine, Wisconsin
48. Kaiser Hospital, San Jose, California
49. Kaiser Steel, Oakland, California and Bristol, Rhode Island
50. Kimberly-Clark, Oshkosh, Wisconsin and St. Catharine's, Ontario, Canada
51. La Crosse Rubber Mills, St. Joseph, Missouri
52. Lockheed, San Jose, California and Los Angeles, California
53. Mays Stores, St. Louis, Missouri
54. Medical Center, Tucson, Arizona
55. Memorial Hospital, Salinas, California
56. Merck Chemical, Rahway, New Jersey
57. Methodist Hospital, Memphis, Tennessee
58. Metropolitan Life Insurance Co., Canada
59. Monsanto Chemical, Rockford, Illinois, St. Louis, Missouri; Muscatine, Iowa
60. Mountain Bell Telephone Co., Albuquerque, New Mexico
61. National Standard Co., Niles, Michigan and Kalamazoo, Michigan
62. National Steel & Shipbuilding Co., San Diego, California
63. Neenab Foundry, Oshkosh, Wisconsin
64. New England Gas & Electric Co., Cambridge, Massachusetts
65. New York Telephone Co., New York, New York and Syracuse, New York
66. Northwood Sawmill Co., Houston, British Columbia, Canada
67. Ohio Industrial Commission, Columbus, Ohio
68. Pacific Telephone Co., San Jose, California
69. Packaging Corp. of America, Cincinnati, Ohio
70. Pennsylvania National Insurance Co., Philadelphia, Pennsylvania
71. Polaroid, Needham, Massachusetts
72. Presto Products, Oshkosh, Wisconsin
73. R.L. Crain, Ltd., Toronto, Ontario, Canada
74. Ratelle Foundation, Columbus, Ohio
75. Republic Steel, Canton, Ohio

76. Rexnord Co., Racine, Wisconsin
77. Rich Products, Inc., Oshkosh, Wisconsin
78. Rockwell Industries, Van Nuys, California
79. Rohm-Haas Corp., Bristol, Pennsylvania
80. St. Mary's Hospital, Racine, Wisconsin
81. San Diego Naval Station, San Diego, California
82. Sandia Laboratories, Albuquerque, New Mexico
83. Schillings Co., Salinas, California
84. Simplicity Pattern Co., Niles, Michigan
85. Stanley Works, Hartford, Connecticut
86. Syntex, Palo Alto, California
87. T.V. Guide Headquarters, Radnor, Pennsylvania
88. Tri-Met Corp., Portland, Oregon
89. TRW-REDA Pump, Tulsa, Oklahoma
90. Teledyne, Mobile, Alabama
91. Textron Industries, Newport Beach, California
92. Trane Co., St. Joseph, Missouri
93. Tranquill Co., Ltd., Kamloops, British Columbia, Canada
94. True Value Hardware, Chicago, Illinois
95. Tucson Medical Center, Tucson, Arizona
96. Union Pacific Railroad Co., Pocatello, Idaho
97. Universal Cyclops, Titusville, Pennsylvania
98. Utica Brewery, Utica, New York
99. Varian Co., Palo Alto, California
100. Vickers & Benson Advertising Agency, Toronto, Ontario, Canada
101. Waterbury & Sons, Oriskany, New York
102. Webster Electric Co., Racine, Wisconsin
103. Western Publishing Co., Racine, Wisconsin
104. Weyerhauser Co., Tacoma, Washington and Kamloops, British Columbia, Canada
105. Xerox, New Canaan, Connecticut

APPENDIX II

*Government Agencies that have Contracted
with YMCAs for Employee Programs*

1. Alexandria, Virginia, Transportation Department
2. Chula Vista, California, Police Department
3. Columbus, Ohio, Police Department
4. Cornwall, Ontario, Canada, Ministry of Transportation
5. Coronado, California, Fire Department
6. Detroit, Michigan, Police Department
7. Des Moines, Iowa, City Employees
8. Duluth, Minnesota, Duluth Transit System
9. Grand Haven, Michigan, Police Department
10. New Westminster, Ontario, Canada, Government Employees
11. New York, New York, Fire Department
12. San Diego, California, San Diego Transit Co.
13. San Dimas, California, City Employees
14. Santa Clara, California, Transportation Agency
15. Ventura, California, Fire Department
16. British Columbia Provincial Government Employees, Vancouver, British Columbia, Canada
17. Wilmington, Delaware, Federal Employees

Workmen's Compensation Agencies
Contracting with YMCAs

1. Compensation Board of Iowa, Des Moines, Iowa
2. Industrial Commission, Workmen's Compensation, Columbus, Ohio
3. Massachusetts Rehabilitation Commission, Workmen's Compensation, Greenfield, Massachusetts
4. Nevada Industrial Commission
5. Ohio State Bureau of Compensation, Cincinnati, Ohio and Middletown, Ohio
6. Oregon State Accident Insurance Fund
7. Industrial Injuries Clinic, Oshkosh, Wisconsin
8. State Compensation Insurance Fund of California
9. Utah State Insurance Fund, Salt Lake City, Utah
10. Workmen's Compensation Board, Houston, British Columbia, Canada
11. Workmen's Compensation Board, Chicago, Illinois
12. Workmen's Compensation Board, Madison, Wisconsin

APPENDIX III

Insurance Companies that have Paid
for Healthy Back Participation

1. Aetna Life & Casualty, Tampa, Florida; Des Moines, Iowa; Phoenixville, Pennsylvania
2. American Mutual Insurance Co., Moultrie, Lousiana and Oshkosh, Wisconsin
3. Aid, Des Moines, Iowa
4. AVMA Group Insurance, Storm Lake, Iowa
5. Bankers Life, Des Moines, Iowa; Storm Lake, Iowa
6. Bituminous Insurance, Des Moines, Iowa
7. Blue Cross/Blue Shield, Salinas, California; Washington, D.C.; Storm Lake, Iowa; Birmington, Alabama; Hyannis, Massachusetts; Memphis, Tennessee; Phoenix, Arizona; Richmond, California; Mobile, Alabama; Butte, Montana; Milwaukee, Wisconsin; Birmingham, Alabama
8. Crown Life Insurance Co., Farmington, Michigan
9. Custard Insurance Co., Des Moines, Iowa
10. Connecticut General, Hartford, Connecticut
11. Crum & Forester Insurance Co., Birmingham, Alabama
12. Crawford Insurance Co., Biloxi, Mississippi
13. Diamond International Paper Co. (self-insured), Cincinnati, Ohio
14. Employees Insurance of Wausau, Oshkosh, Wisconsin and Des Moines, Iowa

15. Esmark, Des Moines, Iowa
16. FMC (self-insured), Pocatello, Idaho
17. Farm Bureau, Mobile, Alabama and Des Moines, Iowa
18. Farmer Fund, Mobile, Alabama
19. Farmers Group, Salinas, California
20. Fireman's Fund, Atlanta, Georgia
21. G.A.B. Business Services, Inc., Des Moines, Iowa
22. Grain Dealers Mutual, Salinas, California
23. Group Health Co-op Plan of Madison, Wisconsin
24. Home Insurance Co., Birmingham, Alabama
25. Homes Insurance, Mobile, Alabama
26. Hygrade Insurance, Storm Lake, Iowa
27. Hartford Insurance Co., Oshkosh, Wisconsin
28. Industrial Indemnity Insurance Co., San Diego, California
29. Insurance Co. of North America, Birmingham, Alabama; Des Moines, Iowa and Salinas, California
30. Insurers Service Co., Birmingham, Alabama
31. Integrity Mutual Insurance Co., Oshkosh, Wisconsin and Des Moines, Iowa
32. John Deere (self-insured), Des Moines, Iowa
33. Kemper Insurance Co., Birmingham, Alabama and Des Moines, Iowa
34. Liberty Mutual, Manchester, New Hampshire; Oshkosh, Wisconsin; Alexandria, Virginia; Des Moines, Iowa
35. Lincoln National Insurance Co., Mobile, Alabama
36. Metropolitan Life Insurance Co., Mobile, Alabama
37. Mission Equities Corp., San Jose, California
38. Moye & Green Insurance Co., Mobile, Alabama
39. Nationwide Insurance Co., Memphis, Tennessee
40. North Central Health Care Plan, Wausau, Wisconsin
41. Ohio Bell Telephone (self-insured), Cincinnati, Ohio
42. Ontario Hospital Insurance Plan, Ontario, Canada
43. Pacific Indemnity Insurance Co., Salinas, California
44. Pacific Telephone (self-insured), San Jose, California
45. Prudential Insurance Co. of America, Mobile, Alabama and Chicago, Illinois

46. R.L. Kratz Insurance Co., Salinas, California
47. Sears Roebuck (self-insured), Yakima, Washington
48. Sentry Insurance Co., Oshkosh, Wisconsin
49. Southern Pacific Transportation Co. (self-insured)
50. Southern Railway Systems, Inc. (self-insured)
51. Sun Life of Canada, Toronto, Ontario, Canada
52. Travelers Insurance Co., Des Moines, Iowa and Salinas, California
53. St. Paul Fire and Marine, Des Moines, Iowa
54. Underwriters Adjusting Insurance Co., Birmingham, Alabama
55. Wausau Insurance Co., Wausau, Wisconsin
56. West Bend Mutual Insurance Co., West Bend, Wisconsin
57. Western Electric (self-insured)

BIBLIOGRAPHY

Walter B. Cannon, M.D., *The Wisdom of the Body*, W.N. Norton, New York.

Thomas K. Cureton, Ph.D. *Physical Fitness & Dynamic Health*, Dial Press, New York 1965.

William Oscar Johnson, "Spray 'em, Play 'em," *Sports Illustrated*, June 15, 1981. An excellent article on Hans Kraus and his approach to sports injuries.

Hans Kraus, M.D., *Backache, Stress and Tension*, Simon & Schuster, New York, 1965.

Hans Kraus, M.D., *Clinical Treatment of Back and Neck Pain*, McGraw-Hill, New York, 1970.

Hans Kraus, Alexander Melleby, and Sawnie Gaston, M.D., "Back Pain Correction: A National Voluntary Organizational Approach," *New York State Journal of Medicine*, Vol. 77, No. 7, 1977.

Hans Kraus, M.D., *Sports Injuries*, Playboy Press, New York, 1981.

Charles T. Kuntzleman and the editors of *Consumer Guide, The Complete Book of Walking*, Simon & Schuster, New York, 1978.

Alexander Melleby, *Jogging Away*, Volitant, New York, 1969.

Hans Selye, M.D., *The Stress of Life*, McGraw-Hill, New York, revised edition, 1978.

George Sheehan, M.D., *Running and Being,* Simon & Schuster, New York, 1978.

Barbara Stimson, M.D., "The Low Back Problem," *Psychosomatic Medicine,* Vol. 9:210, 1947.

Leon J. Warshaw, M.D., *Managing Stress,* Addison-Wesley, Reading, Massachusetts, 1979.

INDEX

Abitibi Price Paper Company, 156
Alternate Leg Lift, 30, 89
Amateur Athletic Union, 150
American Medical Association
   Journal, 147
Arm Exercise, 27

Backache: Stress and Tension, 145
back pain, low. *See* low back pain
Beckmann, Peter, 152
Beecham, Thomas, 130
Bend Sitting, 48–49
Bridges, William, 7

Calf Muscle Stretch, 74, 96, 106,
   118, 123
Canadian Life Assurance Company,
   156
Cannon, Walter B., 149
Cat Back, 34–35, 91
*Clinical Treatment of Back and Neck
   Pain*, 145, 149

Darrach, William, 147, 148
Detroit Police Department, 155

Double Knee Flex, 33–34
Duff, James, 151

Einstein, Albert, 111
Eisenhower, Dwight, 145, 151
ethyl chloride, 147
exercise, 85

failure to exercise, 130
Fetal Position, 21, 90
Fiedler, Arthur, 130
First Hamstring Stretch, 58–59, 93,
   104, 120
flexibility exercises, *see* stretching
   exercises
Floor Touch, 77–78, 97, 107, 119,
   124
flutter kick, 102
full arm circle swing, 103

Gaston, Sawnie, 148, 154

Half Sit-up, 40

ALSO AVAILABLE